BRINGING CULTURE INTO CARE

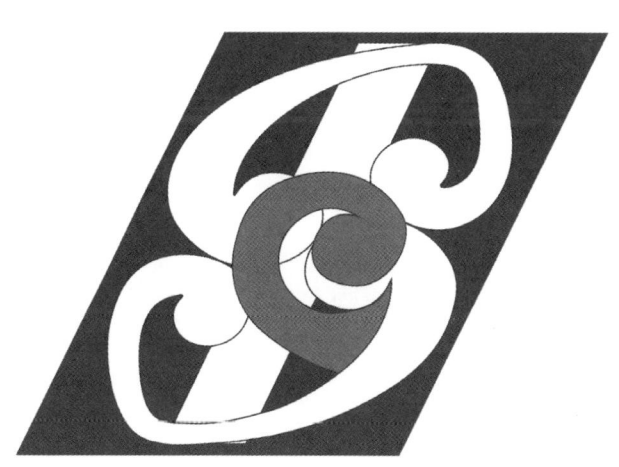

BRINGING CULTURE INTO CARE

A BIOGRAPHY OF AMOHAERE TANGITU

BRADFORD HAAMI

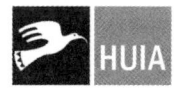

First published in 2019 by Huia Publishers
39 Pipitea Street, PO Box 12280
Wellington, Aotearoa New Zealand
www.huia.co.nz

ISBN 978-1-77550-354-5

Copyright © Bradford Haami 2019
Edited by Katherine Finlayson
Graphic design by Iris Kimberley Murray
Cover image © Whakatane Beacon

This book is copyright. Apart from fair dealing for the purpose of private study, research, criticism or review, as permitted under the Copyright Act, no part may be reproduced by any process without the prior permission of the publisher.

A catalogue record for this book is available from the National Library of New Zealand.

The logo on the back cover and half-title of the book incorporates the original logo for Te Whānau Atawhai services at Princess Mary Children's Hospital, now known as Starship Hospital, Auckland. It was designed by Sam Rolleston. At the centre of the logo is a red koru symbol that represents the development and growth of children. This central koru is supported by four other koru symbolising the four holistic dimensions of Māori health: Te Taha Wairua (the spiritual), Te Taha Hinengaro (the mental), Te Taha Whānau (social) and Te Taha Tinana (the physical). The angled line central to the logo is the manawa or the strength of a person. The whole design is sloped to indicate forward momentum and progress.

This book is dedicated to the memory of:

Mary Hackett (Mary Futter) who was instrumental in opening the door to biculturalism and cultural safety at Auckland Hospital, which resulted in the initial Māori Bicultural Parent Officer position at Princess Mary Hospital.
She passed away in 2016.

The original elders of the Kāhui Kaumātua of Te Whānau Atawhai ki Princess Mary Hospital.

Without all of you, none of this work would have been possible.

Nā Amohaere Tangitu

Hūtia te rito
O te harakeke
Kei hea te kōmako e kō
Ki te uia mai koe ki au
He aha te mea nui ki tēnei ao
Māku e kī atu
He tangata!
He tangata!
He tangata!

If you were to uproot the flax bush
Where would the bellbird sing?
And if you were to ask me
What is the greatest treasure in the world?
I could only reply:
It is people!
It is people!
It is people!

CONTENTS

	Introduction	1
ONE	Karakia and Fish Heads	7
TWO	Ōtākiri	15
THREE	Maternity and Mātauranga	29
FOUR	Confronting the System	37
FIVE	Contrasting Attitudes	49
SIX	Kāhui Kaumātua	61
SEVEN	The Challenge for Dignity	75
EIGHT	Te Whānau Atawhai	85
NINE	Expanding Horizons	97
TEN	Hunga Manaaki	111
ELEVEN	Tangata Whenua Realities	121
TWELVE	Titiro Whakamua: Looking Forward	137
	Appendix 1: Mana Atua	149
	Appendix 2: Photographs	151
	Endnotes	163
	Selected Glossary	173
	Bibliography	175
	Author's Biography	181
	Index	183

INTRODUCTION

Bringing Culture into Care is the story of Amohaere Tangitu, a fearless contributor to the implementation of culturally appropriate care for Māori within mainstream New Zealand hospital practice. This book is a personal account of the struggles encountered by Amohaere and many of her peers who sought the advancement of Māori wellbeing in the mainstream public health sector. Her story reveals how a more culturally appropriate approach to service delivery, known as cultural safety, moved from theory to practice inside the Auckland hospital system and later within other health institutions where Amohaere had a measure of influence to bring about change.

This book stands as an important oral biography of one indigenous woman's career that influenced the breakdown of cultural and racial barriers in the mainstream health system at a time of great political, social and cultural change in New Zealand society. Amohaere is one among many who sacrificed and struggled to challenge and overcome an outdated colonial system she believes was culturally unsafe in order to see culture recognised as an essential part of wellbeing. Her story is only one thread of a finely woven kākahu (cloak) representing the work of many advocates who, with grit and perseverance, pushed for a system of health care that would create better outcomes for Māori. Now that Amohaere has retired (2018), she is able to reflect on the sometimes arduous but satisfactory journey in the health arena where she has made her mark and played her part.

When Amohaere first entered the health system in 1987 as Bicultural Parent Liaison Officer at Auckland's Princess Mary Hospital, it was amidst a period of Māori agitation in the 1970–1980s for social justice and Māori self-determination in the political arena. In the health sector, Māori sought to set in place a more bicultural approach to health care.

From the lowest-ever Māori population level of less than 42,000[1] in 1896, the state of Māori health changed remarkably over the twentieth century. Not only did the Māori population increase tenfold and life expectancy nearly double, but mortality rates plummeted and infectious diseases no longer threatened to destroy whole communities.[2] However, by the 1970s, new health problems began to emerge; mental illness, heart disease and cancer alongside major social and economic upheaval severely impacted Māori health realities.

The concept of what constituted Māori health was significantly revised as Māori sought to transition into health governance and practice that promoted positive acknowledgement of cultural values in the delivery of services. Prior to 1980, Māori were significantly under-represented in the health workforce.[3]

In 1984, the Hui Whakaoranga held at Hoani Waititi Marae in Auckland re-examined Māori health philosophy, discussing in depth the provision and funding of Māori health programmes.[4] In that year too, the Māori Women's Welfare League established a health unit that produced the *Rapuora: Health and Māori Women* report that recommended the establishment of marae health centres to promote primary health care and herbal treatment.[5]

One of the more controversial concepts to be introduced around this period of change was 'kawa whakaruruhau' (cultural safety) – a concept that has now been central to nursing and health worker training for almost thirty years. Cultural safety was designed to bring into nursing education and practice the respect for 'difference' and the recognition of one's own learned personal prejudices that could influence the care given to those of different ethnicities and cultures. It included an emphasis on 'the relationship between nurses, midwives and health service consumers who differ to them by; age or generation; gender; sexual orientation; socioeconomic status; ethnic origin; religious and spiritual belief; and disability'.[6] Deep down, cultural safety addressed the painful issue of race relations or racism within New Zealand health institutions.

During this period of cultural reform, the Auckland Hospital management recognised the need for Māori participation in implementing a more culturally appropriate way of care within the hospital. The bicultural parent liaison role was then created for Princess Mary Hospital, a position Amohaere stepped into. Her main responsibility in this role was to connect with Māori families and communities and identify any cultural sensitivities and issues that impeded care for Māori patients. She continually came up against challenges by Pākehā hospital staff who refused to recognise the validity of her position, many questioning the need even for the existence of her role. Some of her own people labelled her kūpapa (a collaborator) for working inside a non-Māori institution.

Under the Māori initiative Te Whānau Atawhai (the caring family) with the support of Te Kāhui Kaumātua, a pan-tribal eldership, Amohaere carried out Treaty of Waitangi and biculturalism training and implemented culturally appropriate care at Princess Mary Hospital, Starship Hospital and Auckland Hospital. This experience provided her with the expertise that would prove essential for influential change in other New Zealand hospitals.

In 1994, Amohaere moved to Rotorua Hospital as an iwi consultant to ascertain the health care needs and aspirations of the local tribes in the region, becoming Manager Māori Health for Lakes District Health Board. She returned home to Whakatāne in 1997 to carry out a similar iwi consultation and review for Eastbay Health. Here, in 1998, Amohaere was appointed Pou Taratu Senior Manager of Māori Health. She established Te Whānau o Irākewa: Māori Health Services at Whakatāne Hospital and rallied a specialised team of pou kōkiri staff (advanced pillars – Māori health services workers). While this unit took on the responsibility of delivering cultural safety within the hospital service, Amohaere has always believed this should also be the responsibility of all health carers associated with the hospital. Amohaere soon became the Regional Māori Health Director responsible for the overall running of Māori health services for both Tauranga and Whakatāne Hospitals in their delivery of services specifically to the region's Māori clientele.

An integral part of Amohaere's role was to run seminars on contemporary Māori health service policy for hospital staff. This often included giving an understanding of the origin and practical application of cultural safety.

In her lectures, Amohaere would often make reference to a woman's journey through the New Zealand health system from the 1940s into the 1980s. She sought to illustrate why policy and attitudes towards Māori, in particular, had to and did change. This female character encounters racism, prejudice, gender discrimination, chauvinism, violence, misdiagnosis and medical misadventure when engaging with the health system of the day. This woman's journey was often shocking, horrific and almost unbelievable by today's standards of patient care. What most people sitting in these seminars were unaware of was the fact that these incidents were the true life experiences of Amohaere herself.

The contrast between her own unsatisfactory engagements with New Zealand hospitals and the progression of that same system into culturally appropriate care is the main topic of this work. It is also an exploration of the changes in health care for tangata whenua (people of the land) through Amohaere Tangitu's life journey as an agent of change. Amohaere's early experiences with health institutions ultimately armed her with the fortitude and motivation to influence change to a system that clinically had the best intentions in mind for her people but often did not offer any cultural care for Māori. In speaking of her early encounters with hospitals, she says it was an era where 'doctors knew best' and out of fear, Māori people rarely challenged their advice, their integrity or their manner of engagement.

This narrative seeks to accentuate the adverse experiences of Māori and other New Zealanders in a monocultural, outdated hospital system and aims to tell the story of the struggle to find a new indigenous expression of care in the hospital wards. Amohaere's story is not designed to uplift the personal mana of one woman's career journey, and neither is it the intention of the author, nor that of Amohaere herself, to vilify or bring disrepute to the health system. Rather, it is given to bring context and perspectives to the changes Amohaere sought to bring to the system. While this book delves into some deep aspects of Amohaere's personal family life, this work's primary purpose is to highlight how Amohaere and many other supportive peers and elders were able to make effective contributions to instigate change in health care attitudes, policy and practice.

It has been a long-held desire of Amohaere's work colleagues, who have walked alongside her for many years, to produce this book. They insisted her story be recorded to ensure the origin and narrative of her particular 'flavour' of Māori health service would not be lost. In 2012, Amohaere had the title of Distinguished Fellow Māori Health Sciences (Nursing) conferred upon her by Te Whare Wānanga o Awanuiārangi Indigenous University for her outstanding contributions towards developments in Māori health.[7] This event inspired a strong push to see her career recorded in writing. As humble as ever, Amohaere was not fully sold on the idea but has allowed this story to be written after some forceful prompting. Perhaps it was the right time for her to speak now that she has retired.

As an important aside, while Amohaere was known for some time as Judith Tangitu, and then by her married surname of Ngaropo, this project acknowledges that at a certain time in her career she reclaimed her grandmother's name, Amohaere, and later reverted to her maiden surname, Tangitu. For reasons of continuity and to avoid any confusion as to the identity of the subject, the name Amohaere Tangitu is used throughout the text.

In addition to Amohaere Tangitu, I'd like to acknowledge the following people for their essential contribution to the telling of this story: Karena Way, Sir Harawira Gardiner, Phyllis Tangitu, Ron Dunham, Sir Toby Curtis, Dr John Newman, Lani Mārama, Heather Thompson, Pouroto Ngaropo and Tangaroa Ngaropo-Tāwio. Special recognition must also be given to Te Whānau o Irākewa Māori Health Services Whakatāne for support in compiling this work.

Finally, I'd like to pass on my personal thanks to Amohaere for her openness to share her deeper life experiences and views on Māori health with me. I have found her to be a humble heroine who has quietly served her people well. She is someone to look up to as a strong influential leader who deserves honour.

> Mā Ngārangi-o-neherā koe e whakahōnore ou mahi awhi,
> mahi hāpai, mahi manaaki hoki ki ngā hunga hauora me ngā
> uri haumate.

Nā, Bradford Haami, 2018

ONE

Karakia and Fish Heads

The year 1987 was a turning point in the life of Judith Amohaere Tangitu. That was the year she became Bicultural Parent Liaison Officer at Auckland's Princess Mary Hospital. The role, initially unpaid, was designed to create a better relationship between the hospital system and the Māori community, with a particular focus on Māori families whose children had been admitted to the hospital wards. It proved to be an eye-opening experience – not only for Amohaere but for the hospital management and staff as well.

Amohaere witnessed first-hand how monocultural attitudes towards health care and practice, based primarily on a dominant clinical rhetoric – something known by many other Māori working in the system – did not take the patient or their family's cultural or social status into consideration. She believed this system actually diminished the wellbeing of all patients, whether they were Māori, Pākehā or any other ethnicity, by not providing a more holistic health care approach.

'The hospital's code of practice, routines and attitudes were quite often dehumanising,' she recalls.

Her years 'on the beat', walking the wards of Princess Mary Hospital – then the children's hospital – and Auckland's general hospital, saw her witness many practices that were contrary to the Māori worldview and traditions of care. Māori patients and their families often became either highly agitated and unresponsive or simply complied with the treatment, knowing full well the practices were in opposition to their own sense of cultural care.

Māori people also still held a strong attitude towards hospitals as places where people went to die or where families went to pick up their dead. They were not considered places of healing.

'Leave your culture at the door and pick it up on the way out was the common view held by my mother's era,' Amohaere says.

Having an on-site Māori advocate to hear patient and whānau concerns and to bring some comfort into an alien environment brought relief to many. But it also forced Amohaere to confront a huge system about the acceptance of culturally appropriate care. In her cool, gentle but forthright manner, she took these opportunities, not only to serve the cultural needs of patients, but to create an educational environment for staff to experience the fruits of a different approach.

Māori patients had valid cultural concerns that no one understood or cared to do anything about. When Amohaere was approached to intervene, she was compelled to act in a way contrary to standard practice, in the interests of the patients' cultural safety. It was these events that became catalysts for change within the sphere of her pesonal influence.

One pivotal event stands out in her memory. While she was at Princess Mary Hospital, Amohaere was notified about a non-compliant Māori patient at the nearby Auckland Hospital. She promptly walked up the hill and listened to the charge nurse's account of an elderly Māori man who was extremely upset. The nurses in his ward could not understand why he was unresponsive to their care. Amohaere went into the patient's room to find a kaumātua in an incredibly uptight and unhappy state. However, when he saw another Māori face, he simmered down, softened his tone and began to speak openly about his concerns. His strong wish was to have his recently amputated leg returned to him immediately.

With time ticking on, Amohaere approached an orderly – the majority of whom were Māori or Pacific Islanders – to show her where amputated body parts might be taken. 'They're thrown in paper sacks and placed in the big hospital rubbish bins,' was the orderly's response. She asked if he would accompany her to locate this old man's leg, but the orderly, who was Māori, said he was not allowed to do this. 'I won't tell on you,' Amohaere replied. 'You've certainly started something lady,' he retorted, but together they sought out the bins.

Amohaere then asked the orderly to jump in and search the paper bags. He was quite perplexed at her insistence on retaining the body part; this was not normal procedure by anyone's standards. In the end, amongst the refuse, an Auckland City Council paper sack with fresh blood seeping through the surface came to light.

By this time the completely overwhelmed orderly had tried to distance himself from Amohaere. He knew there was going to be trouble. Finding herself carrying the bloodied paper sack through the hospital ward, Amohaere was struck by the realisation that she now had the leg, but what was she going to do with it? 'Did I clean it, wrap it up in bandages and put it in a fresh cleansack? I didn't know!'

She eventually found herself in the principal nurse's office, where the head of the hospital was also present. Fortunately, she had already discussed the matter with Māori community leaders, Dr Ranginui Walker, chair of the Māori District Council, Dr Pita Sharples and Rev. Hone Kaa. Amohaere asked what was going to happen to the leg, explaining that the old man just wanted it back.

'Why?' they wondered.

'Because it belongs to him!'

There was a strong resistance to Amohaere's 'madness'. This was seen as a totally inappropriate request that the hospital or indeed the entire health system could not possibly sanction. The discussion was lengthy as hospital executives sought to understand her cultural position. From her own standpoint as a young Māori woman, she tried to explain as best she could that discarding a body member because it had no more use went against the whole sense of the tapu and mana of the individual.

'From a cultural perspective, a body part is spiritually connected to the whole, and its separation is a cause for distress,' she explained. 'If someone was to mistreat his leg and affect his tapu, he would feel the insult, and this would create a further state of unwellness. If you return the leg, you'll find the old man's wellness will be elevated to the point of early discharge.'

When the heat went out of the discussion, moves were made to settle three issues of immediate concern: creating an environment of healing for the elder; returning his leg in an acceptable manner; and sorting out the best cultural way for its handover without any clinical risk.

Amohaere rang the kaumātua's family to inform them that their elder's leg would be returned. There were tears of elation on the other end of the phone. The family had never thought the request would be heeded and were extremely grateful to her. Hospital history was made when, for the first time, a small casket was crafted to contain the amputated leg, which was held in the mortuary.

Later, the family arrived, backing a station wagon up to the mortuary door in the manner of a hearse. The elders began chanting their karakia (prayer) as they walked into the building. 'At that point I realised this was serious. I took a few steps back behind the orderlies, who were also ignorant of how the procedure was to be conducted.'

The body part had been left in the casket on a trolley in the middle of the room. The elders entered the mortuary with a karanga (woman's call) followed by karakia. They surrounded the casket and whaikōrero (orator's speeches) were spoken directly to it, quoting the leg's genealogy and commemorating the places it had taken the kaumātua. The family then uplifted the small casket, placed it in their vehicle and ushered it back to Northland.

Amohaere herself was met with surprise by the whanāu, who were expecting a kuia. Hearing the surname Ngaropo, they had also expected she must be one of their own Ngā Puhi. Instead, they seemed startled to find a young woman who, they immediately realised, was not one of theirs. This made Amohaere even more conscious of her place as a young woman in this position. The whānau did not warm to her and instead chose to speak directly to the male orderlies about their elder's health. Despite all she had done, intertribal prejudice and gender discrimination were alive and well.

The old man, however, alone and calmed down, set aside his anxieties and began to share with Amohaere about his life.

'Because he was the head of his hapū, as a young woman I was unsure how to approach him and act accordingly. He knew my husband's people and was grateful I had supported him. During the conversation, however, he asked me to ensure his own Ngā Puhi people were present when other Ngā Puhi came to the hospitals. He then cautioned me to seek out the elders.' As far as the old man was concerned, the return of body parts was 'he mahi kaumātua' – the job of male elders, not the work of women.

The kaumātua left hospital with his mana and tapu intact. But the whole episode sparked a wider discussion with the hospital management about the cultural sensitivities and procedures that would be essential for the return or disposal not only of limbs but also of human tissue for Māori patients. Amohaere says that Māori had long been suspicious of how hospitals disposed of body parts.

'This incident also heightened our awareness of respect for the way other cultures like Pacific, Indian and Asian people see health issues and procedures.'

*

Another incident that highlighted the lack of any spiritual sensitivity or cultural competency by hospital workers in the late 1980s happened when, again, Amohaere was asked to respond to a call at Auckland Hospital. This time it was to console an old Māori woman the nurses considered to be uncooperative. Apparently, the old woman kept saying she could see spirits in the room, and she wanted someone to bless it. The staff simply scoffed at her. The nurses felt she should be sent to the mental health patients' ward. They perceived her 'seeing' the spirits of dead people as the rantings of a schizophrenic woman who probably wouldn't live long in her current state.

Unsure of what to expect, Amohaere removed her shoes and walked barefoot into the kuia's room. There, she found the woman softly chanting with her eyes closed. Taking hold of the woman's hand, Amohaere waited for the old lady to realise she was present. Seeing a Māori face, someone who might possibly understand, provided immediate relief to the kuia.

Amohaere didn't see the request for the room to be blessed as at all unusual. Māori always performed blessings and karakia when the realm of death impinged on the physical realm of the living. She approached the head nurse to advocate for the old lady, and a strong debate ensued as to whether or not there actually were dead people in the room. Amohaere thought it didn't really matter what she or the staff believed. Finding a way to return the patient to a safe state of wellbeing was the main issue.

It soon came to light that three people had died in that same room during the previous week, something the kuia had been sensitive to without being told. In this situation, Māori custom would prescribe that a blessing be performed to whakawātea (clear) or whakanoa (make free from spiritual encumbrances) the room. By this time, curious to see the final outcome, the head nurse decided to follow through with Amohaere's request.

As a Catholic, the kuia demanded to have northern minister Pā Henare Tate come and bless her room before she would settle. Amohaere managed to persuade the head nurse, and in due course Pā Tate arrived. After the formal meeting and the karakia, the kuia was satisfied that the dead people were no longer present. Amohaere then asked the kuia if she needed anything else to make her feel comfortable. 'Fish heads would be nice,' came the reply. Again, Amohaere didn't see that as an unusual request.

'I had to go in search of fish heads in the middle of central Auckland to keep the old lady happy. I'd do anything for the elders,' Amohaere laughs.

After searching shops in the city and finally making her purchase, Amohaere walked down the hospital corridors carrying a tray of fish heads and soup, spilling fishy water on the floor along the way and wafting the smell of the delicacy through the ward. This sort of action was unheard of in any hospital in New Zealand.

'The old lady was already up and waiting for her kai when I finally arrived and presented her with the meal. I was elated the old kuia had bounced back to life.'

The karakia and fish heads settled the kuia's mind and heart, and she returned to an amazingly elevated state of health – something the head nurse duly noticed. After two days, the old woman walked out of the hospital as well as could be. The old dear thanked Amohaere greatly for her assistance and her aroha. 'If you hadn't been here for me, I would have surely died,' she declared.

'After this incident, the nurses called me in, accusing me of being a witch,' Amohaere recalls. 'They had all made a bet on the old lady dying.' The kuia's encouraging words spurred Amohaere on to continue in a role that she could see was worthy and lifesaving for her own people.

This event saw a series of further debates and discussions that resulted in new protocols and policies being drawn up for the blessing of rooms where patients had either passed away or were about to. It also paved the way for the first Māori chaplain to be installed in a New Zealand hospital.

*

Practices that prevent the spread of disease-causing organisms are central to modern hygiene, but the notion of hygiene can vary between cultures and genders. Some practices considered good habits in one society can be considered disgusting, disrespectful and even threatening to another.

Medical hygiene is a set of standard practices related to the administration of medicine and clinical medical care. Māori cultural hygiene, on the other hand, is rooted in traditional Māori religious belief and practice. Belief in tapu (sacredness, separation, restriction) played an important role in guiding practices regarding physical and spiritual cleanliness, the sanctity of the body and sanitation associated with everyday living. Karakia was essential to hygienic practice, as was tapu separation. Latrines were removed from the village or home; any form of human waste or body fluid was considered tapu. Cooked food also had the ability to nullify personal tapu and mana, hence cooking facilities were separated from the washing and living areas. Menstruation was the cause for gender separation in some instances, with women not being able to participate in food preparation, gardening or intimate relationships during this period. Childbirth and death ceremonies were highly tapu events that were subject to strict practices of spiritual and physical hygiene and separation from general living spaces.

Māori hygiene standards determined the realms of the living and the dead were never to be mixed. It was considered that this could defile the dynamic of personal tapu and create a state of negative noa (free from tapu) that would diminish the wellbeing of an individual.¹ Māori generally consider wairua (spirit) to be the essence of Māori health. Dr Mason Durie recognises how 'without a spiritual awareness and a mauri (spirit or vitality, sometimes called the life-force) an individual cannot be healthy and is more prone to illness or misfortune.'² Healing is believed to occur at the level of wairua, rather than solely through the treatment of the symptoms of disease. Respect for people and tikanga played a dynamic role in the enforcement of tapu. In the case of violation of tapu, hygiene consequences could occur, hence karakia, ritual practices and removal of the infringement were imperative to create a state of spiritual and physical noa (liberty, freedom from restriction).

Amohaere has always insisted that culturally appropriate care, like clinical care, is not solely a Māori response. 'It should be an approach for everyone, implemented both systematically and personally.' An example of the type of care she so passionately advocates for was illustrated in her own life when an old hip injury began to cause her deep pain. Her original artificial hip replacement had a shelf life of between ten to fifteen years, so in 1992 she opted to have the further replacement performed by a doctor she knew. The cultural conversation with the doctor was interesting. Consents to retain body parts and the relevant karakia were now part of the pre-operation discussion.

'Even though the old hip part was artificial, it still had become part of my body, and I asked for consent to retain it. The hospital agreed. I finally felt safe in the current environment.'

Her own family were part of the proceedings, which began with karakia. On entering the theatre, the surgeon asked Amohaere if she preferred Led Zeppelin or 'Pōkarekare Ana' while the operation took place. Her answer was a given. 'The medical team tried hard to make the sterile environment culturally appropriate for me, which I was grateful for.'

During her recovery, the hospital presented her with a box containing the parts removed during her operation. This would have been a very secretive and tapu subject for the elders to consider in her childhood years, but in this age Amohaere believes that we must be up front about these issues or we will be overwhelmed by dominant views once more and lose our own customary rights and views. Amohaere handed the box to her mother, who took it back to the Rotorua Lakes district, and it was buried at Wahanui urupa (cemetery) at Rotoiti.

Years later, Amohaere had yet another hip operation while she was living at home in Whakatāne. Once again, karakia was incorporated, consent forms for the return of body parts were signed, pillows and flannels were colour coded for the head and posterior – all suitably applied under Amohaere's watchful eye. Her family participated in the procedure by singing her into the theatre, complete with guitar accompaniment. To reduce the sterility of the environment, the Pākehā anaesthetist had created a Māori medley of songs to be played during surgery. 'It was once again a huge difference in the delivery of service. I was certainly comfortable,' she says.

These events provided Amohaere with personally satisfying examples of a total and tangible shift of attitude by health professionals and clinicians. However, in the late 1980s there was much to be done to encourage such shifts.

TWO
Ōtākiri

Judith Amohaere Tangitu's upbringing in a communal environment on a farm at Ōtākiri in the Bay of Plenty holds a special place in her memory. Traditional values such as dignity, hospitality, hygiene, tikanga and respect were everyday concepts central to most Māori family lifestyles in the 1940s.

'Respecting the elders and being of service to the people were two big ethics in our family. Maintaining dignity in life, as well as in death, was another important principle we lived by. These were foremost in the lives of our parents and grandparents.'

These concepts within the whānau dynamic were foundational to the way Amohaere was later to view the application of health care for Māori and for the general public.

Farm life was always filled with people. It was a multigenerational environment with grandparents, grand-aunts, uncles, aunties, parents, children, whāngai (adopted) children, babies and often complete strangers all living together on the same property. On the farm stood a three-bedroomed house with a kitchen and a dining room, an exterior lounge and two separate outside sleeping quarters. There were no electric lights and the wooden floors were covered with potato sacking. The interior of the buildings and the dirt walkways were always kept immaculately clean and in excellent order. There were three baths: one inside for washing bodies, another outside for washing clothes and a third where the corn was prepared for kānga wai (fermented corn). The property supported a milking shed as well as vegetable gardens and a substantial orchard.

Other than her own immediate family of brothers, sisters, Mum, Dad and grandparents, there were many children living in the home. 'Sometimes there were nearly twenty children living in our home at any given moment in time,' Amohaere remembers. As the eldest of her immediate family, Amohaere had the heavy responsibility of caring for the babies and the young children.

'Mum was either working in the fields or caring for the old people. It was a very practical environment, and we all had to play our part. Everyone had jobs assigned to them to keep the home clean. We all had a place to sleep and eat, even if that meant moving out of our beds to accommodate someone else who arrived in the middle of the night!'

The name on the gate of the family farm was 'Rākaupuhi'. This farm was on whānau trust land in Ngāti Awa territory and belonged to the family of her grandmother Amohaere Gardiner (née Powell), who was both Ngāti Awa and Te Arawa.

'My grandfather Tamehana Gardiner worked the land – he was Ngāti Pikiao by whakapapa (genealogy). It was real subsistence living at Ōtākiri in those days. There were sixty acres of land to be worked with rows of garden to be ploughed, seeded and harvested, orchards to be tended and cows to be milked. The entire household would be out in the gardens at the break of day. All of us children would be woken up early to work either in the milking shed or in the gardens. We'd sit on the tractor with Pop as he ploughed up the land. The old kuia with kete on their backs would walk behind in the overturned soil and plant seeds while the children would follow behind turning the earth back over the planted seeds. Kūmara and rīwai were graded and stored traditionally in the rua (storage pit). The children were sent to locate fern to line the floor of the rua for the potatoes and kūmara to be laid upon and covered to maintain a stable temperate environment.'

The produce from the land, with its harvest of fruit and vegetables as well as meat, was all given away to the local families and to the marae when a tangihanga (funeral) or hui (gathering) was in progress. Large supplies of corn, potatoes or watermelons would be left on the front lawn for the local community to come and gather their share of the harvest. This custom is still practised amongst the rural folk in the Ōtākiri–Te Teko region. It was manaakitanga (hospitality) at work. Nothing was ever wasted. Foods were pickled and preserved. Fruits were all made into jams.

There was a mixture of Anglican, Catholic and Ringatū religions and practices to live by and services to attend. The Catholic rosary was recited often, and Sunday hākari gatherings with other local families were common. At other times, the family attended the local Ringatū celebrations on the tekau-mā-rua (twelfth) of each month. There was always karakia in the home for every occasion, including for the administration of medicines.

'The elders seemed to walk freely between a number of religions. All of them played their part, but from memory, the Ringatū prayers entirely in the Māori language were believed to have more power when it came to health issues,' Amohaere muses. The deeper realms of the Māori world were seldom if ever discussed or spoken about around the youngsters. It was more a lived reality, but the finer details of tradition were always carried out with discretion. 'Once I saw them put a coin in one of the sick babies' hands during a karakia session, but I never understood what that was about.'

Healing seemed to be a natural aspect of family life. Cobwebs were left to gather all around the house. 'We were always told to leave the cobwebs alone,' she laughs. When one of the boys cut his leg, human urine was applied to the wound and cobwebs used to seal it. She remembers her grandfather administering medicines. Flax water was for constipation; milk of dandelion was applied to warts; and a dock leaf poultice was placed on boils. Streams of sick people frequented Amohaere's childhood home where the elders administered particular rongoā-a-rākau (medicinal plants) or rongoā-a-wairua (spiritual healing).

Unknown to Amohaere and her siblings until many years later, Tamehana would spend weeks away gathering medicinal plants, then return home to prepare the leaves, bark and roots to create rongoā and bottle and store them in the shed. Although this work was of a secretive nature, Tamehana also recorded all of his medicinal recipes in his private diaries. He'd hand out doses of rongoā when needed, particularly for contraception and sexually transmitted diseases, which had stigma attached to them at that time.

Local tradition held that Amohaere's great-grandmother, Whareraupō, was a healer of mākutu (curses). Her grandmother, Amohaere, was community health-orientated also, and her mother, Mary, had the gift of discernment – knowing where people needed to go for their particular sickness and whether it was a mental or physical illness. Everyone in the small Māori community knew who to go to for specific healing situations. As soon as they saw people coming to visit the home seeking rongoā, young Amohaere and the other children knew to scatter. 'There was an unspoken division between what adult talk was and what was kids' talk. It was all about confidentiality for the visitors and safety for the children.'

Amohaere remembers vividly how automatically the women and children would begin baking bread or puddings as soon as news was heard that a hui or a tangi was to be held at the marae. This mechanical routine has continued throughout Amohaere's adult life.

While her grandfather always donated produce from the farm to the marae, Tamehana never attended any of the local Ngāti Awa funerals in the area. This always puzzled Amohaere, particularly as he would drive down to the marae to pick her up from one. 'I did not know why my grandfather never attended any of the tangi here in Ngāti Awa. Perhaps old tribal rivalries were still very strong then.' While children attended tangihanga, they didn't participate in the formal kawa or protocols of the elders.

'We were never privy to the deeper understandings of Māori tradition till later in our adult years. We were more to be seen than heard. We'd only hear the conversations about healing, life and tangihanga, as well as the noises in the night after dark,' she laughs.

*

The mix of tribal links in Amohaere's veins connect her to Ngāti Pikiao, Ngāti Ranginui, Ngāti Pūkenga, Ngāi Te Rangi, Tūwharetoa, Pirirākau, down to Ngāti Hauā at Waharoa and further into Ngāti Maniapoto. However, living at Ōtākiri, her Ngāti Awa connections were more prominent in the life of the family.

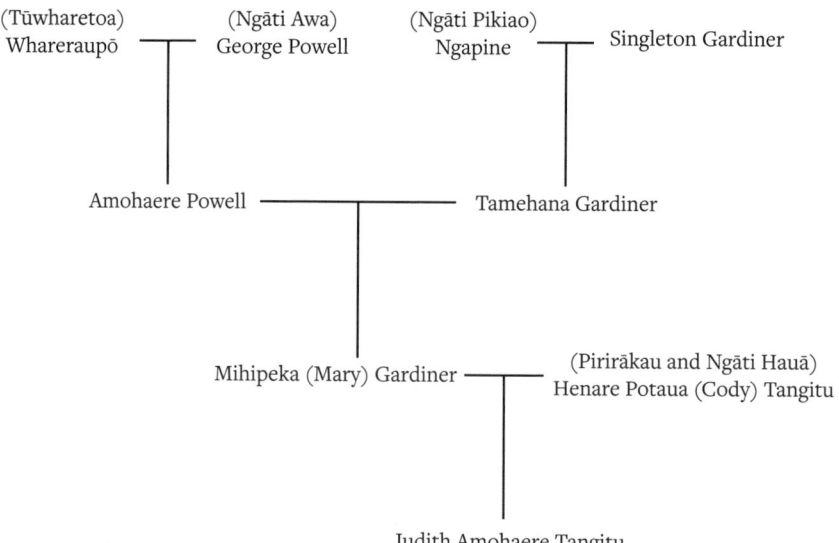

Grandmother Amohaere Gardiner (née Powell) was the daughter of George Powell and Whareraupō Renata of Matatā. She was a dominant force in the family but never overbearing. She attended Queen Victoria Māori Girls College in Auckland in 1910–1911 and later took up mission work at Paeroa with Anglican Minister Rev. John Cowie. She became an active member in tribal affairs and was involved in many organisations during the First World War. She was secretary and treasurer to the Ngāti Tamateatūtahi-a-Kawiti sub-tribe of Ngāti Pikiao and also chairperson of the Waiti Nahue School at Rotoiti. As a service-orientated woman, she was active in helping the local people in the Rotoiti and Te Teko regions, and she was well known for her involvement as an original member of Te Roopu o te Ora – The Women's Health League, under Nurse Robina Cameron (known affectionately as 'Kamerana').[1]

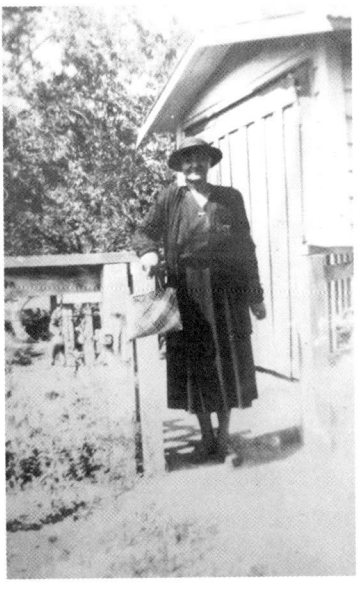

Amohaere's grandmother Amohaere Gardiner (née Powell), a strong woman committed to serving her people.
She was an original member of Te Roopu o te Ora
(The Women's Health League) under Nurse Cameron.
COURTESY OF AMOHAERE TANGITU

The league was actively concerned with infant care, nutrition and housing for local Māori. Under Kamerana's guidance, local women volunteers, often kuia and grandmothers from within Te Arawa, Tūwharetoa, Mataatua and Tai Rāwhiti regions, gave health education to the families of each pā (village). These women also campaigned for the preservation of Māori arts, the teaching of te reo Māori in the schools and a free hospital service.[2] The league was a significant force in the delivery of Māori health services.[3] Later, Amohaere Gardiner became an enthusiastic member of Te Teko Mothers' League.[4]

Her husband, Tamehana Gardiner, Amohaere's grandfather, ran the homestead. He was the only son of Singleton Gardiner and Ngapine of Ngāti Pikiao. Tamehana never knew his Pākehā father; his mother Ngapine's whānau reared him in the old ways. He attended Te Aute College, south of Hastings, and after finishing school, he travelled north to Te Tai Rāwhiti. Here he became involved in land engagement activities inspired by Sir Apirana Ngata, where young men were taught how to work the land and make it sustainable. He then moved back to the Bay of Plenty region as a locomotive driver for the forestry industry. Later still, he shifted to Edgecumbe and Ōtākiri, where he farmed his wife's land.[5]

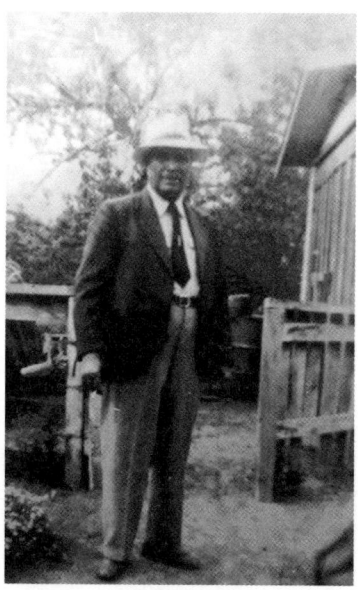

Tamehana Gardiner of Ngāti Pikiao.
COURTESY OF AMOHAERE TANGITU

As a busy member of Te Arawa Trust Board and a number of land blocks, Tamehana was always well respected by the people, in particular his Ngāti Pikiao people. He was a big man, blue-eyed and revered for his: 'Handsome demeanour, cool head and his ability to summarise things up easily. He possessed wisdom and that's why people always sought his opinion.'[6]

Because of the high regard the community had for Tamehana, the police considered his place the first port of call when wayward Māori children needed mentoring, parenting or a temporary home to live. 'Our home was truly communal; we always had new children coming to live with us. I never knew where they originated from, but the police would call my grandfather; he would travel to Rotorua and return home with these children who were state wards,' Amohaere recalls.

Boys picked up for doing something as innocent as stealing marbles were deposited at Tamehana's home, and he had a real heart for these children. Amohaere remembers him reading a newspaper article about some children looking for a home and then driving off to take them under his protection. 'I once saw him drive to Rotorua to pick up a two-year-old and a ten-month-old baby who had been left at home alone for days.'

Young Amohaere never had any trouble accepting the new children.

'We were a mātua whāngai people (parenting and adopting people) established in manaaki tangata (being hospitable to people). There was always plenty of love to go around. We'd carry the children around on our backs wrapped in old army blankets, and I'd have to put them all to sleep as Mum was always busy in the gardens. There was never any distinction between siblings, cousins or strangers – we were all family, all brothers and sisters.'

Love was something seldom spoken of directly but shown in many different ways. 'While we never heard the words "I love you", we knew we were loved; we had a roof over our heads, plenty of kai on the table and clean linen on our beds. That was the elders' way of expressing love. It was unspoken.'

Protection for the children was paramount. Amohaere and her siblings were sheltered from alcohol, violence or crude language to the best of the grandparents' ability. Most of the young ones never saw this side of the world until after they were married. 'There was never ever a harsh word spoken in our whānau as I recall it.' Stay overs at friends' homes were prohibited. The elders didn't trust what might happen to the children once they were out of their sight. The wearing of other people's clothing was also strictly disallowed.

Conversation amongst the older folk was always in Māori, but English was the language of communication to the young people. There seemed to be a parallel universe working within the household.

'The elders and the other families a hundred metres across the road seemed to speak Māori language at all times. For our generation, we didn't speak at all.

My mother was the last of her siblings to be reared with te reo Māori. We were on the cusp of the Europeanisation of Māoridom perhaps. The reo was unintentionally beginning to deteriorate.'

Pākehā ideas of education and language seemed to hold a high place amongst the older people. Pākehā too seemed to be treated differently, especially when they visited the family home. They were treated as if they were somehow superior. The old people had very high standards. 'My grandmother would make sure the house was clean and tidy; she wanted the Pākehā to see us in a good light. There was a very high degree of hospitality afforded them in our home. We'd scrub the table with sand soap, and old Aunty Kiriwera would rub the silverware and cutlery then set the table with the best linen. The old people seemed to move into a whole new level of accommodation when Pākehā people came. Even the elders' English language conversation would be spoken with a type of "plum in your mouth" to fit a presumed Pākehā mould. We, as children, would stand at the door and observe the special kai, language and behaviour, wondering why they behaved differently from their normal home life. That was just their way, I suppose; they wanted to make a good impression with Pākehā.'

The Pākehā world of education was drummed into the young people for the good of their future in the new world. 'We were all sent to school to learn; there was little time to play and become bored.' Amohaere would come home to find the old kuia weaving kete (baskets) or whāriki (woven mats). There was always a big bread and kai cooked with corn, rīwai or kamokamo for the children to eat as soon as they got home from school. There was also a good stock of fruit available from the numerous fruit trees in the fields. 'We'd then be sent up the dirt tracks to gather mānuka for brooms.'

*

The traditional system of tapu and noa, strictly observed in the home, dictated the way hygiene and cleanliness was administered in the whānau. Men and women bathed separately. Because of a shortage of tank water, everybody would wash in the drains. The men would always wash first, then the women. Waters were never shared between men and women; the elements of the genders just could not mix. Anything to do with the disposal of human body waste was tapu and always carefully considered and dealt with. Human waste as well as hair and nails were an extension of a person and still possessed the hau o te tangata (personal vitality), which if meddled with, could diminish one's wellbeing.

Towels for the body and tea towels were never mixed. Tea towels were soaked in the copper, but towels for drying the body were washed elsewhere. Clothing was scrubbed and washed down at the drain with the clothes being rubbed against the large nearby rock. Anything to do with hair or the body was never to be anywhere near food or the kitchen. Clothing associated with sleeping and bathing towels were prohibited from the kitchen or dining area. Anything associated with 'below the waist' was highly tapu and respected.

The time of the mate-mārama, a woman's menstrual period, was extremely tapu. Women were unable to go swimming or to participate in any food gathering, garden work or eeling during this time. In a previous era, women had a separate dwelling area away from the main tribal living space where they lived until the menstrual period was over. 'When I had my first period, many things changed. My clothing changed, I could not mix with men, even my seating changed. I could only sit in specific places now.' Amohaere was in a transition time in her life. 'I didn't really understand what it was all about. The padding used to deal with women's menstruation, I was told to leave in the shed outside the house. These were later gathered by the old kuia and secretly disposed of during the night. I never knew what the old people did with these things.'

Sex was even more of a secretive subject. 'It was sacred, even tapu. I was always confused how people learned about sex in those days; we were so ignorant.' Amohaere's mother was a Catholic and she would ask the local priest for information on certain subjects. 'She would return with a book for us youngsters to read on sexuality rather than speak to us directly.' Marital bedrooms were also considered tapu; children were never allowed access without permission – it was definitely understood to be a couple's private space.

'Everyone in the household seemed to know the automatic rules around respecting each other's boundaries. These days the plans for building houses are totally void of understanding cultural values associated with cleanliness and hygiene; bathrooms, washrooms and toilets are often stationed right next to the kitchen or dining rooms. This is totally against traditional Māori sensibilities.'

*

One of the old people Amohaere fondly recalls was Aunty Kiriwera. She was a cousin to Tamehana and lived in a little cottage on the farm. The old kuia had been ill-treated in her life and was very unwell. Tamehana gave her a place to stay till the end of her days.

'Aunt Kiriwera was a unique-looking woman. She had a shrivelled-up body, was hunched over, had teeth like tusks and a beard. She knew little, if any, English and often spoke to herself as well as to the cats, dogs and all the other animals. We'd all tease her as she shuffled along, but I loved her. She had the mind of a five-year-old and lived in her own world.'

In today's world, Kiriwera would probably be assessed as someone with 'special needs'. In those times, Māori communities cared for their own at home with whānau. These included people who would be identified today as traumatised, wairangi or pōrangi. This was in contrast to the western psychiatric tradition of confining people with a mental health condition or intellectual disability away from society as if they were contaminated or even, in extreme cases, denying their existence.[7] Despite their state of mind or quirky ways, these whānau members were just part of the family. No one would have ever thought of putting them in a home to simply waste away. Kiriwera with her unusual ways was just part of the whānau dynamic.

'I'd see her weaving whāriki and washing our clothes on the rock. She was an enigma from an older world. I'd lead her around the property wherever we needed to go. She'd shuffle along in her shoes; she was just part of our everyday life.'

In Kiriwera's little cottage was everything she owned, which wasn't much. It included a small old tin Amohaere always marvelled at. 'This tin contained rings she had made herself from the silver tinfoil paper inside the cigarette box packaging. It was ingenious.'

Praying the rosary was always a tedious task for the young family members. Amohaere found it monotonous to sit still and recite and listen to the rosary. Often this prayer time was held in old Kiriwera's cottage. For a time, Amohaere had her bed made up next to the old lady. 'My mum and my grandparents didn't want her to be alone.' It was during an all-night rosary prayer time, with all the children present, that Amohaere's mother informed them that old Kiriwera had actually passed away. 'It wasn't the first time I'd had to face death as a youngster,' Amohaere says. 'My mother had lost twins, so we had to be with them at that time as well. Death never frightened me.'

Amohaere and her mother were charged with cleaning and dressing Kiriwera. 'My mother went and got her a new set of clothes and left me to bathe the kuia. I still remember her in her pink nightgown. When the body dies all the fluids and excrement pass out, so this needed to be cleaned first. I remember not being scared at all; it seemed so natural for me to do this work. I remember her skin was so wrinkled but so very soft and her feet were pink.

When my mother came back, we talked to Kiriwera as we moved her body in any way and apologised as we washed her private parts. There was a sense of urgency in what we had to do before rigor mortis set in. Together we dressed her, and I brushed her hair so she would look beautiful.'

Amohaere was then stationed to sleep by the dead kuia's side to keep her company until the family came to take her to the funeral director or to the marae. She wasn't to be left alone. 'I loved her. I was never afraid of sleeping next to her whether she was alive or dead; there was nothing to be scared of. It's the living you need to be careful of my mother would say. She taught me to respect the deceased; they had dignity too, you know. That was the first time I had bathed a person who was deceased. It's a caring call to dress dead bodies, but my mother taught me to respect both the living and the dead.'

The next day, the undertaker arrived and old Kiriwera was carried from her bed to the hearse as the karanga (woman's call) rang out. She was then taken to Rotoiti where she was buried with whānau.

This was an incident, like many in Amohaere's life, that prepared her for a yet unforeseen future in health.

*

Healing, sickness and death are natural states that each society deals with in its own way. For the local tribe, seeing a doctor required trust. It was not so much they doubted the doctor's clinical or professional knowledge, it was more about how comfortable the relationship between them would be.

'I heard the elders speak of Dr Golan Maaka of Whakatāne. He was a former Te Aute College student from my grandfather's era, and the people really trusted him,' Amohaere remembers.

Dr Maaka was a medical practitioner well loved by the local Ngāti Awa and Tūhoe people. He created a more welcoming environment by running his practice from his own home. Here, people would be less intimidated and more accepting of western health methods. The people had a strong relationship with him, most on a first name basis.

Dr Maaka's knowledge of whakapapa, the local people's histories, and especially his familiarity with the people's cultural sensibilities allowed for a more open medical exchange, a better assessment of the health problems and a responsive attitude to treatment. 'Dr Maaka created an accommodating environment where Māori was spoken and Māori values were uppermost. That was a big thing that earned him trust,' Amohaere says. 'The tribes all gathered at his house at Whakatāne and sat around his property as if it were a marae.'

He was a doctor who recognised both the world of western medicine and the spiritual world of the Māori. He understood as a western-trained doctor how he could work medically to bring healing, but he also knew what illnesses needed to be referred to the local tohunga Māori. There was no judgement in his decisions but more of an acceptance of the two often opposing value systems. 'The old people more than respected him; they loved him,' Amohaere remembers.

The hospital system was another kettle of fish. One of Amohaere's first experiences with any kind of state care occurred when her father, Cody, had a debilitating road accident. The Gardiner home was a respectful place where harsh words and violence had never had a foothold. 'It was my father who brought violence into the home. Very little was spoken about it, and I never understood why.'

There was a viewpoint held by Pākehā and Māori of that era that you choose your bed and you lie in it. This seemed to be the discourse that strongly prevailed, and it was certainly the view held by Amohaere's grandparents towards their daughter Mary who had married Cody Tangitu of the Pirirākau tribe of Te Puna, Tauranga. Their relationship was fiery. Cody was an adventurous daredevil who displayed frustration and agitation at times, while Mary was vivacious, philosophical, stable and the glue of the family. She was also a matakite (seer). However, their relationship changed dramatically.

It's a story Amohaere tells reluctantly. 'My father was in a coma after an uncanny accident. He was never the same and had to be admitted into the mental health care system. It was so sad.' Amohaere was fourteen at the time; Cody was thirty-six.

For a while, Cody had been a sharemilker at Te Puna until he changed occupation and returned to Ōtākiri where he became a top forklift driver at the Tasman Pulp and Paper Mill. He often had to work double shifts, and on one occasion, on his way home from Kawerau, he had a motorbike accident on the Te Teko–Edgecumbe road next to Kokohinau Marae. The accident was so severe that he was in a coma for six months in Whakatāne Hospital.

'Hospitals were considered a no-go zone by families in those days. They believed it was a place to go and die; a place of kēhua (ghosts).' This was a valid cultural belief considering the hospitals of the time were purely clinical, and cultural and spiritual values were never factored into health care. Māori very rarely spoke about their fears; it was more of an unspoken conviction, and as a result, people tried to fix a health issue themselves rather than go to the hospital. Often the hospital was a last resort, and by then, it was too late.

Local people had their own ways of caring for health and that included seeing the local tohunga for remedies. 'In my father's case, he was sent to hospital to his deathbed, but he did eventually recover. After coming out of the coma, he was released and we brought him home, but his brain had been adversely affected.' The extent of his brain injury was not fully revealed till he returned home. 'He was always agitated, angry and constantly delusional, living in the past. No one had any real idea of the impact the continual deterioration of his behaviour would have on the family.'

Worried for the whānau, Amohaere's grandfather Tamehana took Cody to the local tohunga searching for a specific Māori healing. He sought additional opinions from the local Māori doctors as well. Sadly, no one was able to return Cody to full health. Hospital doctors reassessed his situation and decided it would be better if he was admitted to Tokanui, a large mental health institution near Te Awamutu. They were insistent he was dangerous and that he had to be committed. 'My dad's behaviour became more erratic and agitated when he realised what they wanted to do; he didn't want to go. I remember the moment the ambulance drove up our driveway.' It was the first time Amohaere had seen medical restraints in action. 'Men in white coats wheeled out a trolley with all sorts of straps tied to it. They then had to restrain him with a straitjacket; that's what the assessment said. He had to be checked into the local hospital in a straitjacket. It was heartbreaking.'

Amohaere was appalled by the health staff's treatment of her father. To her it was just 'plain bad'. Cody was later transferred to Tokanui Hospital by Tamehana and Amohaere's cousin and foster brother, Wira Gardiner. The catchment area for this hospital included the Bay of Plenty and reached as far south as New Plymouth and was probably why Cody was transferred there. 'He was medicated to the limit and kept behind bars for years,' Amohaere says sadly. 'I never knew why he was treated like that.'

Cody was released from Tokanui in 1993. 'Dad couldn't really come home, so he was sent to a residential home in Matamata.' On a visit to Matamata with her mother, Amohaere was horrified to find her father in a cockroach-infested room with a mattress on the floor in the corner of the cold basement of the home. 'Sadly there was nothing we could do.' However, in the end, the whānau brought him home where he lived for an additional eight years, with Amohaere's sister. 'We tried to look after him, but he was never the same. It was hard work, but we kept him home till he died.'

Cody was in state care for almost forty years. 'The hospital care I witnessed then seemed the complete reverse of what I was brought up with; it was cruel and offered patients little dignity.'

Amohaere's experience of the health system, particularly with her father, made the prospect of working in that sector the last thing that she would ever want. However, destiny was to have its way. Māori women were already earmarked to become nurses, and Amohaere would be no different. In addition, coming, as she did, from a lineage of ancestors who had healing in their hands, her calling and that of other whānau members may have been set more by providence than by freedom of choice.

THREE

Maternity and Mātauranga

Amohaere attended Edgecumbe College and was that school's first Māori prefect. However, she did not pass University Entrance, and her grandfather urged her to train for a job. She applied to be a kindergarten teacher and even had a reference from the Ngāti Awa paramount chief Eruera Manuera, but she didn't make the grade. She then tried her hand at nursing. During her training, she was sent to the Kawerau maternity home for three months on practicum before further training at Whakatāne Hospital.

'My grandfather had great hopes for me. But I never completed the nursing training, which disappointed him no end.'

Grandfather Tamehana then took her to Papakura to sit an entrance test for the army. This was successful, but her grandfather's hopes were again short-lived, for it was here that she met a young man, Samuel (Sam) Ngaropo, and fell in love. He was Ngā Puhi and Ngāti Awa – in fact they were distantly related.

Amohaere's relationship with Sam was not sanctioned by Tamehana and other family elders. 'My grandfather was most upset as he had organised an arranged marriage for me, which I was not interested in at the time.'

It was not long before their first child was on the way. When labour pains reached a certain stage, Amohaere knew she had to go to the hospital. She was accompanied by Sam and her mother, Mary, who was extremely excited by the arrival of her first mokopuna (grandchild). The birth seemed normal, but there was some apprehension because the baby was premature. When he was delivered into the world of light, he was cleaned, wrapped up and briefly shown to Amohaere before being rushed into a separate room and placed in an incubator. At that stage, there was no indication from the staff that anything was wrong.

It wasn't until the next day that the ward staff wheeled her newborn son in to her on a trolley. He was wrapped up with his eyes closed. A little flower had been placed on his body. The nurse announced to a shocked Amohaere that her baby had unexpectedly died. It was Christmas Day 1966.

'I could hear my mother and Uncle Te Rame Raerino outside in the hallway exchanging strong words. They were arguing about where the baby would be buried. Mum wanted him to be buried at Tapuaeharuru Marae and Uncle Te Rame wanted him to go to Umutahi at Matatā. At the time, I was so ignorant of those types of things. I was just in complete shock.'

To console her, the nurse told Amohaere they had called the local Catholic priest during the night to the child's bedside where he had administered the last rites, baptising the baby with the name John. This was all sanctioned by the hospital but performed without the mother's consent.

'In shock, I wasn't too upset about this at the time, but I certainly never asked them to name the child.' Amohaere's right as the parent to name her own baby had been taken away from her.

In addition, she was refused the right to be discharged by the hospital. At that time, a maternity patient could not leave hospital for fourteen days, and despite numerous requests, Amohaere was unable to attend her own baby's tangi and burial at Umutahi Marae.

'I was bereft because I was denied the right to mourn and enter into the traditional mourning process. The only saving grace in this situation was the fact that I was home, close to my mother and whānau.'

Visiting a city hospital during her second pregnancy the following year was just as degrading. Having now shifted to Herne Bay in Auckland, Amohaere needed to go to St Helen's National Women's maternity hospital for a standard prenatal check-up. She made the trip reluctantly and alone. Sitting in the waiting room, she found herself surrounded by Pacific Island women whose understanding of English was limited. The hospital secretary's pronunciation of waiting patients' Māori and Pacific names was deplorable. When Amohaere's name was called, she was greeted at the door by a very stern Pākehā nurse who ushered her into a room. 'Her demeanour was just plain bad,' Amohaere remembers.

She was ordered to strip off and put on a standard hospital gown with an open back. 'Most young Māori suffered from whakamā or shyness, especially when it came to revealing our bodies publicly. Here I was, alone with just a light gown wrapped around my body and not really knowing what to expect.'

The nurse led her to another room and instructed her to lie on a sterile examination bed to wait for the doctor. When Amohaere asked for a covering or something to warm her body, the impolite nurse rummaged through the room and threw a blanket at her. Amohaere felt the nurse's bad attitude was due to her being unmarried and Māori.

'It was as if she was sniggering about how stupid these unwed mothers are, especially these dumb young Māori women who find themselves pregnant so young.'

Amohaere tried to cover her body down to her knees and waited patiently for the doctor to come and check that everything was well with her baby. After a while, a male doctor accompanied by a team of trainee doctors, all men, entered the room. They all wore white coats and had stethoscopes dangling from their necks. The nurse had vacated the room, leaving the young woman alone with these unknown men. The doctor's attitude was similar to that of the nurse. He looked Amohaere up and down as if to say, 'Here's another unwed Māori mother.'

The doctors talked amongst themselves. There was no eye contact with Amohaere. They all stood at one side of the bed and stared as she was ordered to disrobe. They touched, probed and gawked at her naked body without an iota of direct communication. Amohaere felt it as a blatant invasion. In her upbringing, no man was ever allowed to look upon the woman's nakedness unless they were husband and wife. She lay quietly, tears rolling down her cheeks. No one seemed to care about how this young mother-to-be might be feeling. Not one question was asked of her. The men talked to each other and wrote on their charts. When they were done, they simply left the room, still ignorant of the effect of their uncouth manner on a shy young patient.

'I was just a learning session to these white men. I felt I had no dignity left.'

Ashamed and perturbed, Amohaere slowly got dressed and, still crying, vowed she would never endure a hospital examination again. She declined further invitations for regular check-ups.

The next time she went to the hospital, again alone, was when she was in labour. There were complications. The baby was born prematurely, weak and in need of medical attention. He was briefly shown to his mother then taken out of the room.

Later a nurse wheeled Amohaere into the recovery room where the baby was struggling to breathe. 'Would you like to have a priest come?' Amohaere was asked. 'Why?' she replied. 'Because he will die soon,' the nurse replied. This baby was named Samuel Tawio Ngaropo, and he lived for only one day.

'I rang home and relayed the sad news to my mother, who immediately said they would come up to take the baby home for burial.' Little did she know that Sam had made other plans to bury their child at Māngere Cemetery. When Amohaere's mother arrived from Ōtākiri, she asked for the baby. 'I watched her face drop when she heard he had already been buried in foreign soil. She didn't agree with Sam's decision, and what's more, he had no idea he had done anything wrong.'

Once again, Amohaere was unable to leave the hospital to attend her own baby's burial. It was also heartbreaking looking on while women in the same room were giving up their childen for adoption when she had just lost a baby that she desperately wanted to keep.

'To make the situation even worse, there was a sense that the child's death was somehow my own fault for not attending all the health checks. That was even more hurtful.'

When she was discharged from hospital, Amohaere demanded that Sam take her to where their baby was buried. 'When we arrived at the cemetery we could not find him. Sam couldn't remember where our baby Samuel was buried. I couldn't quite believe what we were going through; it was so sad.' In fact, the baby had been buried in a pauper's grave with a number of other children. 'I lamented deeply. I couldn't cope with it. It just didn't ring right with me.'

Losing her two baby boys in consecutive years was a huge grief for Amohaere. Many years later, the whānau returned to Māngere Cemetery to uplift baby Samuel and return him to Whakatāne. The cemetery managers could not locate where he was buried. 'I walked that graveyard until I found him myself. It was just a mother's instinct; I knew he was there. We found adult corpses had been buried over the top of the babies. There was no way we could return him home. What a debacle. Instead, we compromised and took soil from that gravesite back with us to Umutahi.'

These events surrounding childbirth were not exclusive to Amohaere. Many New Zealand women, both Māori and Pākehā, were treated in the same manner. Amohaere's experiences were a sad echo of her own mother's maternity hospital ordeals, which were never spoken about. These issues had been too painful and too secretive to reveal. Mary had had three sets of twins who all died of blue baby syndrome, a heart defect where oxygenated blood mixes with non-oxygenated blood, causing the baby to turn blue and eventually die. All Mary knew was that her children died as blue babies, and she had never had the condition explained to her by doctors or nurses. The added heartbreak with the first two sets of twins was the fact the babies' bodies were never returned by the hospital to the whānau. To this day, no one has been able to find out where they disappeared to once they had been taken out of the delivery room. Speaking with other Māori who suffered in the same way, this seemed to be a standard practice in hospitals at that time.

The third set of twins to be born and pass away were returned to Amohaere's parents to be mourned and then buried with proper protocols at the Matariua urupā at Te Teko. 'My mother was filled with internal grief at the loss and removal of her babies,' says Amohaere, who deeply empathises with her mother's grief. 'She was so suspicious of hospitals and always felt they had stolen the babies to study them. And this was all done without her formal consent. The hospitals had total control, and we, the people, had limited say over our own bodies and families.'

With Amohaere's third pregnancy, things were again touch and go. Still unmarried, she did not feel she could go to a hospital. Nevertheless, a Plunket nurse came to visit her four times. Each time, she was refused entry despite insisting that Amohaere keep the appointments for her baby's sake.

'This nurse wanted me to trust the system, which I certainly did not, but I was so unwell at the time I relented and did as she said.' Eventually, Amohaere began to trust this persistent nurse who made regular visits to check her progress and accompanied her to the new St Helen's Hospital.

'The Plunket nurse stayed with me right up until the child was born; she was a real rock of support for me,' a grateful Amohaere remembers. At seven months, the premature baby boy arrived. He weighed five pounds and was immediately put into an incubator. Even on this occasion, Amohaere thought the doctor's attitude towards her was less than caring.

It was only after the safe delivery of this first surviving son, Nicholas Ngaropo, that Amohaere and Sam married at Sacred Heart Church in Vermont Street, Auckland, in September 1968. The young couple went on to have three more healthy sons: Samuel, Christian and Tamehana.

*

The young family soon found themselves embedded within the community whakapapa of those Māori families living in Te Atatū North, West Auckland. This enclave of pan-tribal Māori families was made up of those who had shifted to the urban cityscape due to the pull towards 'work, money and pleasure' and the push of the unsustainable earning power of their rural multiple-owned tribal lands.[1]

The Māori community here rose dramatically from a population of only 125 to 766 between 1956 and 1966. Melissa Williams writes how Te Atatū North 'consisted of pioneering Māori leadership and collective Māori activity that assisted in the overall long-term development of Māori West Auckland'.[2] This saw the establishment of a Māori language day-care centre, Māori committees, Māori culture clubs, the erection of urban marae such as Hoani Waititi Marae and the rise of the urban Māori authority Te Whānau o Waipareira Trust.

While there was plenty of work available, Māori workers were exposed to a system controlled by the pressures of a cash-driven society, which had no regard for Māori communalism or culture. Government policy sought to integrate Māori into a so-called 'normal' Pākehā way of life. Underpinning this and previous assimilation policies was the idea that being Pākehā would be the saving grace for Māori. Being Māori had no place in the new order of New Zealand life.

Amohaere and Sam's marriage was certainly tested in this environment, with one partner (Sam) believing in the mantra that 'being Pākehā is better' and the other striving to maintain 'being Māori'.

Amohaere had to raise her sons in a volatile living situation fuelled not only by these conflicting philosophies on life but also by alcohol. She didn't drink and had never witnessed a lifestyle governed by alcohol in her own upbringing. The impacts of this nakahi nui (great snake) among Māori grew as Māori urbanisation increased, especially with hotel opening hours being extended from 6 p.m. to 10 p.m. from 1967. Drinking had become a normal, legitimate and socially tolerated activity, and the bar room or local tavern became a substitute marae for many urban Māori. Amohaere and her young family, along with many other urbanised Māori families, bore the brunt of these substitute norms and their impacts.

It took courage for Amohaere to step out of her own hidden home life to engage with the outside world. She took the opportunity to work as a cook at Te Atatū Tavern and later at Penfold Wines. The simple job of cooking fish and chips for the punters became a kind of lifeline for Amohaere. Drunk or sober, the people loved her cooking.

Later, she applied for a position as a cook at the local children's group home where young people with behavioural problems were cared for as state wards. These Social Welfare homes were created by the government to house delinquent and deprived children. In the 1980s, there were twenty-six institutions, disproportionately filled with Māori children – a population that had grown steadily since the 1960s.[3] Amohaere was a witness to the high percentage of Māori children in this group home in Te Atatū North, which was run by Pākehā managers. The children were considered to have behavioural problems, but many were at risk or had been abused in their own dysfunctional home environments.

The children seemed to be drawn to Amohaere, always fronting up to come and peel spuds and kūmara (sweet potatoes) with her in the kitchen. The kitchen became the perfect environment for conversation. She'd ask them their family names and where their whānau originated from. This became a point of connection as Amohaere knew many of the family names. Other staff were intrigued to see how the Māori children seemed to be attracted to Amohaere and engaged with her in a different way.

'I suppose I seemed like a nanny to them. These children were missing something of their own identity.'

Amohaere had always dreamed of serving her own people in some way, and cooking for the children in the home had awoken that moemoeā (dream).

'I looked at the children and asked the question: what could we do differently for them rather than bringing them into a world of bad parenting skills, sexual abuse and violence? I had a passion to make a difference not only in my own home but in the lives of these children.'

*

At this time John Rangihau (Chairman of the Māori Advisory Council) and John Grant (Director General of Social Welfare) came to review the home with a view to closing it down. They were both part of a Ministerial Advisory Committee on a Māori Perspective for the Department of Social Welfare that produced an influential report called *Puao-Te-Ata-Tu (Daybreak)*, in 1986.[4]

There had been a growing awareness that these types of homes were unsuitable for most young people, and moves to close them down began in the mid-1980s. It was recognised that the needs of the large number of Māori children in these institutions could not be met by management and staff and that other action was needed for their future care. The committee's report noted its belief that the Department of Social Welfare was a highly centralised bureaucracy that was insensitive to the needs of many of its clients.[5]

The report also mentioned the 1984 Māori Advisory Unit Report from the Auckland regional office, which had expressed grave concerns about institutional racism in the department and its rules that reflected the values of a dominant Pākehā society.[6] At the heart of these issues, the committee believed there was a 'profound misunderstanding or ignorance of the place of the child in Māori society and its relationship to whānau, hapū and iwi structures'.[7]

John Rangihau was adamant that the children needed to find their identity and make connections back to their wider tribal families.

Before the home was closed, Amohaere organised for the children to visit a number of marae in the eastern Bay of Plenty to help them understand something of their own culture. This trip saw them visit Tapuaeharuru Marae in Rotoiti, Tūterēinga Marae at Te Puna, Kokohinau at Te Teko and Kauae Tangohia Marae at Waihau Bay. Most of the children had never visited a marae let alone slept inside a whare. It was a learning curve for all of them, and many made whānau connections they had never previously known about.

John Rangihau had been surprised to find Amohaere as the home's cook. He knew her family lineage well and convinced her to go to Carrington Polytechnic for training in social work. He also felt her education should be paid for by the state via the children's home. 'He was very concerned that the system needed more qualified Māori in this sector, and he really influenced me a lot.'

When the conversation about Amohaere's desire to study arose at the children's home, the manager insisted this was not an option for her. He thought she would be better suited as a cook for another home they had already planned to transfer her to. Defiantly, Amohaere applied to study for the basic papers in the Community Health Certificate at Carrington, and despite the home principal's opinion of her potential career options, her entry was accepted. Amohaere remembers being the only Māori in the class of that year with a Dutch woman as the main lecturer.

During the course, Amohaere learned about the state of the nation in relation to drugs, alcohol, violence, general and mental health, housing, abortion, youth pregnancy, suicide, prisons and community services. Māori life expectancy was lower than non-Māori; the Māori unemployment rate was 14 percent as opposed to non-Māori at 3.7 percent; Māori incomes were far lower than non-Māori; and Māori comprised 50 percent of prison admissions.[8]

The explosion of mātauranga (knowledge) that Amohaere soaked up while she was at Carrington led her to ask more searching questions as to why her people were in this sad state. In some ways, it reflected her search for answers to her own life circumstances. The combination of the often tragic incidents with so-called hospital care, her personal family circumstances and the realisation of the huge social disparities between Māori and non-Māori were to become a springboard for a new trajectory in Amohaere's life. She was determined to find a way to make some kind of a difference in the lives of Māori.

FOUR

Confronting the System

When Auckland's Princess Mary Children's Hospital advertised for a Māori parent liaison officer in 1987, Amohaere promptly applied. The successful applicant would be responsible for helping families through the whole experience of being in hospital.[1] Establishing a better working relationship between the hospital, Māori patients, their families and communities was also essential to this role.

Over the years, hospital staff had noticed that Māori children being admitted to the wards would, more often than not, be unaccompanied by family. They noticed too that Māori families seldom visited their children or mokopuna, despite nursing staff making strenuous efforts to reach the patients' kin. Māori children were also constantly returning to hospital with preventable diseases. These were real concerns for hospital management, and something needed to be done.

In 1985, the Auckland General Hospital Principal Nurse, Mary Futter, had come to realise that hospital staff were 'missing the point' when it came to caring for Māori patients and being culturally sensitive to their needs.[2] She recognised there were cultural differences at play. No matter how conscientiously hospital staff cared for clients clinically, too often an unsatisfactory outcome for Māori seemed to prevail. It was apparent to her that the biggest obstacle to a bicultural understanding of health care was the monocultural attitude held by the hospital policy makers. Putting the focus on patients' needs rather than those of the health providers and identifying racist attitudes both in the health system and personally were crucial to changing the status quo when it came to treating Māori.

Mary Futter first became aware of racism in New Zealand in 1978 when she witnessed the army and police forcibly remove 222 people from Auckland's Bastion Point, Ōrākei, after a 506-day occupation protesting against the continued loss of supposedly inalienable Māori land on this block. Besides becoming politicised to the reality of the Māori–Pākehā divide, she was deeply challenged about how to support Māori within her own sphere of influence.[3]

Nurse Futter approached Bob Scott, then Director of the National Council of Churches Programme on Racism, to ask how she might help educate hospital management and policy makers on these issues. This was the start of 'talking about education on institutional racism'.[4]

Later, further efforts were made to seek Māori advice about how to walk down this path. Nurse Futter sought out Auckland University academic and Māori Council chairman Dr Ranginui Walker and former Race Relations Conciliator Peter Sharples for their views. Both advised her to employ Māori within the system, working in the area of Māori services. This was imperative if the system wanted a favourable response from the Māori community with better health outcomes as the goal. A Māori liaison position was mooted.

Prior to appointing a Māori liaison officer, however, it was strongly recommended the hospital implement an acceptable anti-racism education programme to pave the way for whoever took up the job. There was concern that a lone officer would just 'die under the stress' of the enormity of the role, due to the size of Auckland Hospital and the large number of Māori entering the wards. At a meeting in 1986 between Race Relations Conciliator Wally Hirsch and Bob Scott, it was agreed that dealing with the issue of institutional racism would be an essential requirement.[5]

As a result of these discussions, the Auckland Hospital management group agreed to employ a project worker to implement an education programme with the following objectives:

1. enable clients to participate in decisions about personal health in accordance with their cultural tradition

2. ensure those delivering health care have regard for cultural values of individual clients

3. ensure policies, procedures and systems of the hospital are designed to recognise and cater for the needs of all cultures.[6]

Karena Way, a Pākehā race relations educator, was interviewed for the project worker position accompanied by a support team of twenty-five Māori, including Titewhai Harawira, who had also arrived on the scene to support

Karena. This sent whispers throughout the wards that Māori activists were taking over the hospital. When Karena was employed in mid-1987, hers was the first position of its kind in New Zealand health. She only agreed to take the job if the hospital management team first underwent the training to show their public commitment. It took nearly two months before that agreement was forthcoming. All three members of the management group – the Medical Superintendent, the Hospital Manager and the Principal Nurse, had to agree equally for this bicultural training and vision to be accepted.[7]

Under extreme pressure, a lack of office space, no phone and open discriminatory acts against her, Karena organised and ran seminars for the management group and all department heads. Many of those invited to attend did not turn up. Others left angry and confused when confronted with their own racism, while the majority made drastic shifts in their perceptions. Strong criticism and hurtful racist comments rose to the surface, but once it was explained that the seminars were aimed 'at an institutional level and not at individuals personally', people's fears subsided.[8] The hospital management team of the time were in total favour of walking this way delicately as they saw the future value in the bicultural approach to aid provision of the best possible standard of care for all patients and their families.[9]

*

Institutional racism (known also as structural discrimination) was described in the 1986 *Puao-Te-Ata-Tu* report as 'the most destructive and insidious form of racism' where national structures are rooted in 'values, systems and viewpoints of only one culture'.[10]

Racism was recognised as a key determinant of negative health outcomes and further polarisation between Māori and non-Māori. The term 'institutional racism' was commonly used to describe the bias inherent in organisations controlled by Pākehā delivering services to an over-represented section of the Māori community.[11] One definition of racism describes it as an attitude or an ideology 'that accepts racial superiority, and, when present in those with power, justifies them using that power to discriminate against and deprive others of what is rightfully theirs on the basis of their race'.[12]

Institutional racism is considered difficult for organisations to recognise internally as it can occur unintentionally. Informal practices embedded in everyday organisational life effectively become part of the system, becoming unequivocably 'this is how we do things around here'. One of the aspects of institutional racisim that the Human Rights Commission recorded as needing to be addressed in this era was 'medical care and rehabilitation services that fail to account for different health needs and values of different communities'.[13] Hospitals in New Zealand had traditionally embraced English-based values to the point that 'there was little difference between a hospital in England and one in New Zealand.'[14]

Puao-Te-Ata-Tu called for a more conscious effort to make our institutions more culturally inclusive in their character and more accommodating of cultural difference. The report pushed for 'change to penetrate to the recruitment and qualifications which shape the authority structures themselves'.[15]

Education on the topics of anti-racism, biculturalism and the Treaty of Waitangi was needed to facilitate general acceptance by hospital staff of the coming changes in policy and practice. This was in line with government changes of the time where entities like health boards were to become state-owned enterprises that would be required to act in a manner consistent with the principles of the Treaty of Waitangi.[16]

The Treaty became a focus for New Zealand race relations in the context of Māori economic, social and cultural development.[17] In a paper delivered to the Royal Australasian College of Physicians' annual scientific meeting in Wellington in 1988, Dr Mason Durie identified the recognition of the Treaty as having major implications for the future maintenance of Māori wellbeing.[18] He highlighted how the New Zealand Standing Committee on Māori Health had recommended in 1985 that the Treaty articles 'be regarded as the foundation for good health in New Zealand'.[19] Then in 1986, the Department of Health recognised the Treaty of Waitangi as having 'special significance' and supported the statement that Māori concepts of health, officially recognised under the Treaty, and appropriate services for Māori had a right to be funded through the nation's health system.[20] In 1989 Dr Mason Durie envisioned a future partnership between New Zealand health workers and Māori:

> It would be misleading to minimise the impact of Western health practices or the contributions they have made to the health of Māori people. Clearly, what is needed, however, is more evidence of a genuine partnership between tribal elders and health professionals each acknowledging the other's relative authority, their worldviews, and their limitations. Health workers will continue to bring new technologies and treatments. Tribal leaders will be aware of the wider dimensions of health and the importance of relationships between healthy people, land, the environment and cultural integrity.[21]

Getting to this place would mean a major institutional and attitudinal shift.

One incident that compounded the situation of seeking change in hospital attitude and practice occurred when a Māori mother discharged her child from urgent care at Princess Mary Hospital. When this mother entered the hospital barefoot, poorly clad and carrying a sick child, she was treated with disdain by staff. She took offence and left the hospital with her child. Without proper clinical care, the child later died. Contact was made with the hospital's principal nurse Mary Futter[22] over this situation. She responded by helping to force open the door to cultural recognition and practical change in Princess Mary Hospital. She was certainly a visionary.[23]

These types of incidents were a recurring theme. Taking into account the consultation with Māori and the challenges presented by the anti-racism education programme, the appointment of a Māori parent liaison officer was now considered to be essential. Karena Way still had to dissuade hospital management from employing a Pākehā with strong Māori community associations to fill this position. She believed management needed to support Māori in these sorts of positions.[24]

The job was advertised and published in the newspaper in te reo Māori. It was indicated that interviews would also be conducted in Māori. Amohaere was interviewed by the Auckland Area Health Board team, which included Janet Jackson (Divisional Nurse Manager of Paediatrics), Rev. Eru Potaka Dewes (Auckland District Māori Council Chairperson on Health) and Joan Head. Amohaere's uncle Toby Curtis stood in support of her application and sat through the interview alongside her. In the selection process, hospital management thought Amohaere's particularly quiet nature was an asset[25] as opposed to an aggressive activist type who might upset the status quo. Amohaere was offered the position and began her career in Princess Mary Hospital on 14 September 1987.[26] There was no doubting this would be a deeply political position.

*

The liaison role was round the clock on demand, supporting Māori patients in the wards and connecting with families in the community. It was intially only a voluntary role – until an honorarium or koha could be organised. It would be two years before a full wage would be allocated to Amohaere's position.

There was no orientation process for Amohaere. She had to find her own way around the eight wards in Princess Mary Hospital and learn to weave her way through the halls of power in the organisation to build a rapport with the staff. Nobody knew what powers the bicultural liaison position really had, what it actually entailed or its relationship to other staff positions. There was probably little, if any, appreciation for it. Amohaere would have to flesh out the routine and mechanisms herself and work out how best to carry out this role.

Her ignorance of the hospital system made it an even more difficult road to walk. There was obvious resistance in the organisation to her presence. Statements like 'not another Titewhai Harawira' were hurled at Amohaere – a reference to events that were unfolding at the Wharenui Unit and then at the Wharepaia section of Carrington (psychiatric) Hospital.

It was a totally foreign system. Amohaere describes it as 'sterile, cold and so very unwelcoming'. Doing her rounds was fraught with an array of racial attitudes that would take a courageous type of person to tackle. Old memories came flooding back to her, but now she would encounter that hospital system as an insider – a system based completely on clinical care.

'There was no regard to creating any kind of close rapport with patients, their families or taking into consideration the cultural values of Māori and other people,' she recalls. These were not part of any curriculum taught to up-and-coming doctors and nurses.

'What are you – a doctor or a social worker?' some staff enquired bluntly. There was no legitimate box in which to place her position. One of the heads of child health was particularly sceptical. 'He held an invisible gun at my head, speaking directly at me, asking "What do you think you are going to change in this place?" It was certainly an "us" (Māori) and "them" (the hospital) mentality.' Other Māori and Pacific Island staff also saw Amohaere, the newcomer on the block, as a threat. 'Who does this woman think she is? That was the attitude I gleaned even from the brown staff,' Amohaere reflects. 'I just had to stand my ground.'

A large part of her position was to ensure incoming Māori patients were made to feel culturally comfortable in the hospital environment and to allay possible non-compliance. Initially, Amohaere reported verbally to Janet Jackson. Later written reports were required. 'Janet knew well the purpose of my role. She trusted me and never looked over my shoulder.'

For Amohaere, seeing sick children was never pleasant, but the opportunity to see them recover and leave hospital was always a true blessing. Understanding why Māori families were not visible as visitors for their children was paramount to both Amohaere's position and the hospital's obligation to tangata whenua. There was a prevailing attitude fostered amongst hospital staff that Māori were uncaring and abusive towards their children. Amohaere believed this was certainly not the case with all Māori.

Travelling with the district nurse to visit families of children in hospital opened her eyes to the lives of Māori living on the poverty line. The state of many of these homes was atrocious. Trying to communicate with families about their children was almost impossible as the district nurses found it extremely hard to create a rapport with them. 'Māori would see Pākehā come to their homes and whakamā (shyness, shame) would arise, and no contact would be made,' Amohaere explains. The nurses, doctors and hospitals didn't know how to create a connection with Māori families and their communities. There was also little desire to engage. 'Approaching a house, I'd see the curtain open and then close. Seeing a Māori come to the door, our people were at least a lot more open to receiving us.'

Visiting these homes was a sad affair. Often no one in the household was employed; there was no income to buy food or furniture and certainly no way to travel into the city. 'I would get stuck in and clean their homes and work out a plan whereby the parents could come and be with their babies. As far as the parents were concerned the children were already being cared for with the best attention and food at the hospital.'

Amohaere remembers a baby coming into the hospital in need of a heart operation. What caught her attention was the fact that there was no family member accompanying the child. Often parents wishing to be with their sick children had nowhere to stay close by and were governed by hospital visiting rules. In those days, families were only permitted to come into the wards during specific hours. This was just not possible for poor families out in the regions who had large families to care for back at home. The rules made it extremely complicated for them to be present as a comfort to their child in hospital.

It didn't take Amohaere long to realise the obvious; there was no accommodation available for parents and whānau who needed to be close to their children. Because health providers were practically non-existent in the regions, families had to travel long distances to visit their children. Often one or both parents worked night shift, and they were unable to visit at all. Other times, families had no money for the petrol needed to make multiple visits during the week. Amohaere strongly maintains that these situations were by no means a picture of Māori parents' lack of love for their children but more the consequence and pressure of circumstance.

Amohaere would arrive at the hospital at 6.30 a.m. and find parents sleeping in their cars or later find they had waited in the wards for hours to see their children. Hospital administrators and staff would walk blindly past them, ignorant of the social and economic condition of these Māori families. 'This issue was right on the hospital's doorstep, but no one could see it clearly.' Families were known to park in the Auckland Museum grounds to sleep in their cars, using the public toilets and the lily ponds, filled with goldfish, to wash. When visiting hours arrived, they would walk into the hospital. There was little money for expensive parking fees, and more often than not, families would incur multiple parking fines.

Sometimes mothers would hitchhike from outlying districts as far away as Papakura, Pukekohe and Waiuku to visit their children. They would have no clothes, no petrol, no food, no money, nowhere to sleep and no friends or family to connect with. It was often a very foreign world. 'One mother approached me in the corridor asking me for money to go and visit her six children back in Pukekohe. People were torn and desperate. It was heartbreaking to see.'

Follow-up was crucial to creating a relationship with these families. Often Amohaere would drive the mothers home. Months later, she would receive a letter or card thanking her for her kindness. 'Many of these people would cry and wait for me to appear in the wards just to have someone to talk to who actually showed some care. That's all they wanted.'

Amohaere could see families were in dire straits and struggling to cope in the modern urban world away from close-knit whānau. 'There was no such thing as health providers in the communities and certainly no iwi, hapū or marae involvement in these people's lives. Everything was centralised, and that was problematic for them.' This, she says, produced unsafe environments for Māori children. It was imperative that parents be by their bedside for the healing process. 'The hospital had no idea what the issues were that kept families away. We just simply had to do something.'

At staff meetings, Amohaere would report on the state of visiting families and why most could not be at their child's bedside. Dr John Newman, one of her initial antagonists, believed the hospital needed to put something in place for families. He introduced Amohaere to the board, where the chairman asked what it was she wanted to say. Addressing the board for the first time, she felt nervous and out of place as she told them of families staying near the lily pond. 'We will consider your views,' she remembers the chairman responding. A vacant ward was made available as family accommodation.

'It certainly was a celebration when this accommodation became a reality. We named this space the Whānau House.' It was a major breakthrough. The premises were hastily cleaned up, furnished, mattresses delivered, curtains hung, a kitchen resourced and a living space created for visiting families.

Amohaere has fond memories of her introduction to the Friends of the Hospital, an influential group of middle class wealthy women who raised funds for the hospital, headed by Dame Rosemary Horton. 'They were initially ignorant of the realities of working-class families when I came to speak with them.' But Amohaere was able to share with them about the need for creating a space for Māori and other families to stay close to their children.

These women were deeply touched, and with tears, they honestly recognised their ignorance about the social and economic circumstances of Māori families. 'There is poverty in our midst!' This comment made by one of the Friends still resounds with Amohaere.

The Friends became Amohaere's greatest supporters in campaigning for an accommodation facility close to the children's hospital. She salutes them. 'They may have looked upper class, but they were down-to-earth caring people. They were instrumental in organising food and brand new or unused clothing to be sent to the new accommodation for visiting families.'

Some of the elders from Mataatua Marae in Māngere, including Brownie Williams, Aronia Ahomiro, Tamihana Thompson and others, volunteered their time at the Whānau House as kaumātua to welcome families and to care for their needs. These elders, along with Amohaere and other hospital workers, created a roster to stay on site and receive family members who would turn up late in the evening or early in the morning. Amohaere believes that without the support from these folk, this kaupapa would never have survived.

As soon as the Whānau House opened it filled up quickly and additional needs became apparent. There were Māori, Pākehā and other groups who would seek a place to lay their heads – it was open to anyone. House rules stated that families paid a koha (monetary gift) for their stay of whatever they could afford. 'Poverty was huge out there, people didn't have much. They would arrive with their loved one on an ambulance without a change of clothes or money to buy food.' Volunteers sought resources from companies, which donated canned foods and breakfast cereals, while individuals donated clothes from their own homes to the Whānau House. The facility became a godsend for hundreds of families.

News of the Whānau House at Princess Mary Hospital spread like wildfire. Auckland's general hospital was very interested in Amohaere's smart modification, and it wasn't long before the need for a similar facility there became a critical reality.

That moment came when a well-known Tūhoe elder from the Bay of Plenty was admitted to Auckland Hospital accompanied by near-on a hundred whānau members demanding accommodation. When the hospital could not provide this, the whānau expressed strong feelings that this was just not good enough. Māori news media were called to investigate why the hospital could not provide accommodation for family members, many of whom had travelled a great distance. Staff were highly agitated, not knowing how to handle the situation. Amohaere and the nurse manager were notified of the growing tension.

When Amohaere arrived at the ward, she was confronted by an angry crowd not slow to show its contempt. As a Māori within the establishment, she was subject to a tongue-lashing. As calm as could be, Amohaere put a call through to Koro John Turei, a Tūhoe elder living in Auckland. He promptly arrived, and his relations were pleased to meet with one of their own. Meanwhile, Amohaere and hospital staff had to face reality. 'We disscussed the issue and everyone knew this whānau weren't going to move, so it was agreed to search for an area where we could house them. That was a better idea than the continued conflict.'

Ward 7 in the general hospital was identified as temporary accommodation, and in a short time, mattresses were laid out and facilities prepared to sleep up to a hundred people. There was relief in the air, but the situation was short-lived as the kaumātua passed away during that night. Despite the heavy confrontation, Amohaere did get appreciation from the family, some of whom returned to thank her personally weeks later.

A similar incident occurred when a well-known Ngā Puhi family arrived on the scene with a sick relative. Once again, there were harsh words and complaints about the lack of facilities to house Northland whānau. Again, Amohaere and the nurses were called to the scene. 'While the family were surprised the hospital had a Māori liaison system in place, yet again I was grilled about not fulfilling their will and catering for their needs. We had to find another space to accommodate these people. They weren't going away any time soon.'

Having married into Ngā Puhi and carrying the Ngaropo name made things even worse for Amohaere. 'So you're not one of us?' was the implied accusation. Despite the verbal abuse, Amohaere and the nursing staff found a ward where fifty people could sleep temporarily.

'All the tribes were on our back. Staff would ask me how I could handle the abuse, and my answer was always the same: "We're Māori, and we know how to work things out."'

It was obvious to Amohaere that hospital staff were extremely afraid of Māori and their aggressive approach to these types of affairs. They did not feel equipped to deal with people management, anger or cultural issues. With hindsight, this scenario had been an issue for years and didn't just affect Māori families. 'While I was an advocate for Māori first, I never isolated myself only for Māori, but [I was] for Pākehā and anybody else too. It wasn't just about Māori but the general respect for the wellbeing of all patients and their families. But my obligation was to Māori first.'

Reports of these incidents reached the ears of the decision makers at senior management level. Amohaere was invited to share her views and offer her solutions. In time, Auckland Hospital was to create a Whānau Room that provided accommodation for families, initially free of charge, based on the same principles as the Princess Mary Hospital Whānau House. This was a real breakthrough in the New Zealand health system at the time.

These accommodation units did not come about easily; they took a lot of negotiation and time. Many of the whānau that frequented them arrived with their normal home habits, which sometimes put the validity of these spaces in jeopardy. A security guard rang Amohaere one night about a raging drunken party in the Whānau Room, giving her the heads-up before the police were called. The family's kuia was in hospital, but the whānau of three who were offered the space to stay in had instead decided to gather all their urban relations to have a party. Amohaere stormed the building to find a crowd of thirty people seated on beer crates in a smoke-filled room, tossing back alcohol. Sternly, she sorted the situation out, and the whānau were whakamā, not realising the ramifications of their behaviour. Amohaere was not judgmental. 'They were only doing what they know and how they have always acted. We have to just accept the state some of our families are in and engage with them where we can.'

As with any new concept, there is bound to be a period of trial and error. As a result of these sorts of incidents, tighter management constraints were put in place but not so heavy as to chase families away. Today, Auckland's Starship Hospital supports Te Whare Awhina, which provides short-term accommodation primarily for whānau who live outside the Auckland region, while local Auckland families supporting an acutely ill patient are considered on a case-by-case basis.[27]

FIVE

Contrasting Attitudes

The attitudes of Māori towards hospitals and the opinions of hospital staff about Māori have been detrimental for Māori health in general.

Historically, the interaction was complex. The poor distribution of hospitals meant restricted access, owing to long distances from Māori rural communities.[1] Discriminatory hospital policies and a reluctance to admit Māori who could not pay their fees became further barriers.[2] Some Pākehā are said to have actively discouraged Māori participation, while Māori often believed hospitals were exclusively for the treatment of Pākehā.[3] Many Māori became disillusioned with western medicine, while others actively sought hospital care.[4]

In a paper written for the 1959 Young Māori Leaders conference, Doctor Golan Maaka of Whakatāne elaborated on Māori apprehension about modern medical methods. He observed that Māori were reluctant to visit nurses and doctors or enter hospitals due to a suspicion of Pākehā methods, fear of tapu infringements and the belief that only the tohunga could cure a particular Māori disease.[5] He further commented that Māori attitudes to modern practice began to change because of the dramatic results of antibacterial drugs, modern surgery and the untiring efforts of district nurses and medical officers in the preventive field.[6] Speaking about the local Whakatāne region, he noted that Māori would still attend the empirical treatment of the tohunga, after receiving modern treatment, 'just to make sure and look after the Māori side'.[7]

Amohaere shares: 'In my mother's day when the people entered the hospital, they would automatically leave their reo (language) and their tikanga (protocols) at the door. They believed there was no wairua (spirituality) in the hospital, so they'd say, "When you leave this place pick them (their tikanga, wairuatanga and reo) up on the way out."'

These beliefs rose to prominence in response to a hospital environment that did not accept any other way of administering care except the Pākehā way. This, Amohaere believes, led to Māori disregard for general and emergency hospital care, with many patients deciding to sign out in an unwell state only to be re-admitted later in a more critical condition.

Walking the wards, Amohaere became more acquainted with the hospital organisation and its day-to-day running. She quickly became aware of practices that were in opposition to Māori views about hygiene. She and other colleagues saw it as their responsibility to bring these issues to the attention of hospital management. One alarming example of transgression of cultural hygiene, pointed out by Amohaere, Karena Way and others to hospital management, was the situation of the exterior docking bay and the way it was managed. The single dock behind the hospital was where incoming food products, goods and medical supplies entered the hospital. That same dock also served as the single exit for outgoing hospital rubbish, toxic materials, dirty laundry and linen, as well as human body parts. This dock was also where the tūpāpaku (dead bodies) were transferred out of the hospital.

This mixing of the realm of the living with that of the dead was a transgression of Māori hygiene standards. From a Māori perspective, the notion of having incoming fresh food meant to nourish living patients crossing paths with outgoing laundry, daily rubbish and, in particular, tūpāpaku was unhygienic, to say the least, and cause for the contamination of food and medicines. It also diminished the mana (reputation, authority) of the deceased. This contamination was then imparted to those who partook of the food and medicines. It was considered this situation could defile the dynamic of personal tapu (sacredness) and create a state of negative noa (without restraint or restriction) that would diminish the wellbeing of a person.[8]

This activity was not in the public eye, so who would know this was occurring? Those patients or family members sensitive to the metaphysical world would detect the defilement as cause for further unwellness. Amohaere would hear hospital patients complain of passing dead bodies in the corridors or of sensing the spiritual contamination of foods or linen. Secretly, the patients would request karakia or a chaplain's blessing.

Once hospital management, and later Māori elders, was informed, management was forced to make changes. Senior staff, food services, funeral services and contractors would all have to be informed and educated on the changes. Plans would need to be made for renovations. The flow of internal and external traffic would have to be re-routed. Blessing the pathways that tūpāpaku took through the wards would have to be instituted and new building plans actioned. Dealing with this situation meant a policy change and was by no means a small task; it took time and the release of funds to make the change a reality.[9]

The hospital was a world of its own. Consumer participation in health care or the notion of patients inquiring, commenting on or being involved in medical decision making was practically unheard of prior to the mid-1990s. Doctors or nurses did not ask patients for their personal points of view. Discussions about tikanga or cultural difference, the consent to return body parts or placenta, the relevant touching of people and the tapu of flannels, pillows and bedding were simply not on the radar. The subject of an alternative way of care for Māori was definitely challenging for clinicians and staff, considering only the clinical perspective ruled[10] and the dominant medical premise of never compromising clinical care was as strong as ever.

From the outset in her position at Princess Mary Hospital, Amohaere says she felt a hardness of heart by staff towards Māori. Prevailing attitudes were grounded on stereotypical and uninformed observations rather than a more intimate knowledge of the people, their ways and their social circumstances. Amohaere perceived how health workers often labelled Māori as aggressive and uncaring towards their children. They were criticised as drunkards, constantly ridden with alcohol-related diseases, diabetes and rheumatic fever and over-represented in sexual abuse cases. They were also portrayed as non-compliant hospital patients. These attitudes and beliefs were reflected in the way nurses and doctors treated Māori patients harshly, as if their illnesses were their own fault and they needed firm and even stern treatment. Comments like 'Maybe the Māori disposition to bad health was cultural, biological or even genetic' or 'They deserve what they get' were commonly expressed sentiments. Others believed Māori were 'genetically wired' for aggression.[11]

*

A patient's first impression of the hospital is often reflected in their initial interactions with nurses. 'Nurses did not have good communication skills with Māori; they were ignorant of Māori and Pacific languages and were known to yell at patients if there was a communication breakdown,' says Amohaere. Nurses came across as very stern and considered themselves always correct.

In turn, Māori stayed quiet and never spoke up. There were never any of the formal greetings Māori people were used to in everyday life. There was no reo or tikanga-based engagement. Patients and staff who spoke other languages were reprimanded or made to feel inferior and out of place if they were heard speaking their mother tongue. English was considered the only language for communication in the wards; all others were regarded as foreign langauges, including te reo Māori, which had at that time, only recently been designated a national language of New Zealand.

Where nurses and doctors could not understand the language of patients in the wards, janitors or orderlies who could understand were asked to interpret. Often inadequate translations would be given in answer to specific questions, and this sometimes resulted in inappropriate medical care. At other times, old kuia would speak their language to Māori-looking doctors or nurses only to become whakamā (ashamed) when it was realised that they could not understand.

From her own training days, Amohaere remembers the matron's instuctions to young nurses to never touch a patient. 'You don't hug them or relate to them; that is not your role. Your role as a nurse is to take their pulse and that's that.' There was never any move to create a relationship with patients, but simply to perform the clinical procedures. It was a very sterile world.

Traditionally, nurses were educated not to recognise people's differences in the provision of nursing care. However, recognising difference and challenging the unconscious negative attitudes nurses may have had towards difference were going to be imperative for quality care. This was central to the notion of cultural safety, a concept originally developed by Irihapeti Ramsden and the Nursing Council of New Zealand.[12, 13]

As stated earlier, many of the hospital practices were blatantly adverse to commonly held Māori views of hygiene and tapu. Māori were culturally conscious of maintaining a separation between an individual – especially the head, which is regarded as tapu – and anything associated with food, bodily fluids, other people's body parts and death. These were elements that could nullify the personal mana and tapu of an individual. In dealing with patients, nurses would place soiled bedding, bedpans and urine bottles on food tables and lockers during cleaning sessions. Pillows designed for the head were used for other parts of the body, while beds where patients had recently died would be immediately allocated to new patients without any form of blessing or whakawātea (removal of any residue of death). Bandages, tweezers and other surgical utensils would be sterilised and constantly reused. Limbs and pito (umbilical cords) were not returned to patients or families despite continual requests.

Doctors would touch the head of a Māori patient without consent – a sacrilegious act in Māori eyes. Some doctors received a stern rebuke from elders for this though they were usually none the wiser as to the cause for the reprimand. Similarly, male doctors and specialists touched women's bodies without seeking their consent. 'This was so common. I'd raise my voice to the medics and ask "Would you let your mother do that to you?" They'd always reply "No!"'

Most doctors saw the extended family members gathered in the hallways or bedrooms as a nuisance. Whānau would be asked to step away from the patient as doctors wearing their white coats, stethoscopes, masks and gloves would make their examinations. Medical jargon was the norm, with little or no plain explanation of the clinical findings offered to either the patient or family. Confused family members interested to understand their loved one's diagnosis or prognosis would sometimes seek out Māori or Pacific orderlies or even tea ladies to find out what was happening to their hospitalised whānau. There was a reluctance by clinicians and nurses to pass down vital information to family members.

'While standing with one whānau as their son was being examined by seven doctors, I introduced myself and explained to the doctors this was the boy's family. I could feel their resistance. They all nodded, but there was no real response to my request to be there.' Later, a doctor approached Amohaere on her rounds and asked her for help in that same boy's room. Doctors had been blocked from examining the patient by the family surrounding their boy's bed and refusing to move.

'I went in and hugged the kuia of the whānau and the rest of the family. She told me how she was not comfortable with the way the staff had treated them all as if they did not exist. I told the kuia she must stand up and have her say, rather than stay passive.' The kuia then spoke directly to the doctors about the mistreatment of her family in no uncertain terms. She certainly had their attention as Amohaere made a quiet exit. 'I wanted our people to stand up and say something. They didn't have to take that kind of treatment.'

Amohaere considered Māori to be too compliant towards doctors and nurses – sometimes to their own detriment. There was an attitude that Pākehā doctors and nurses knew how to fix Māori. This was part of a wider national belief that doctors were to be trusted as they knew everything. On the other hand, Māori would very rarely speak up, question or challenge what they were being told, or how they truly felt. It was frustrating for nursing staff, who would often complain that 'they never say anything'.

Māori were generally shy people with a strong respect for elders and those in authority. This was a cultural norm in Amohaere's day. It was common for the people never to fully speak up clearly to doctors about their illnesses or answer questions clearly because of this cultural reality of respect. They would simply agree with whatever the nurses and doctors would diagnose and accept the medication given to them without question. 'In many cases, due to the lack of full, comprehensive communication betwen patients and doctors, the people's ailments were often misdiagnosed and wrong medication was administered.'

As an advocate for Māori patients Amohaere was always privy to their concerns. Family and patients often did not feel they could openly share because they believed they would not be listened to. It seemed to her that children in the hospital didn't have a voice and neither did their families. She remembers one Māori mother speaking up on her son's behalf about insensitive treatment by the staff, only to be told to be quiet. 'Meanwhile, the Pākehā nurse continued to take her unsympathetic attitude out on the child, who was constantly crying. No one would say anything about the mother's concerns with this nurse's racist attitude, so I spoke directly with the principal nurse about this situation. This caused havoc as my presence opened up a whole new can of worms.'

'I was so naive in those days. I'd lie in bed at home wide awake all night thinking about how I was going to find the best way to work with racist attitudes. I had to be careful I didn't internalise my own personal attitudes against the system or Pākehā and take it out on the patients like this nurse did.'

Hospital processes were often very exclusive, and staff were often uncommunicative. A child being seen in the acute ward could only be attended by specialist staff. Families were required to wait out in the corridors away from their loved one, often with little or no communication as to their child's progress. 'Being inclusive, I'd continually update families as to what was going on and what their child's progress was. This was something the families appreciated greatly.'

Parents felt safe meeting Amohaere. It was her intention to ensure the family felt they were in a comfortable environment with qualified staff who understood their ways and, most importantly, that their loved ones were in good hands. 'I was committed to visiting the patients regularly. I didn't want the whānau to be in a hurry to leave their child's bedside.'

A head of the pediatric hospital apologised to Amohaere once for his and his fellow doctors' behaviour. He realised there had never been any training on caring and understanding patients in this way. 'You are opening a door for us, Amohaere,' he said. They hugged, and from that time, Amohaere says, he began to realise what biculturalism really meant. He would seek her out whenever he needed to talk about tikanga Māori issues. 'I knew the doctors and managers needed evidence to prove my points before they would consider any form of change.'

Dying and deaths of Māori patients tended to spark particularly difficult and unpleasant interactions between staff and whānau. When doctors tried to obtain consent from parents to perform post-mortems, collective discussions with wider whānau proved problematic.

On one occasion a man was rushed into hospital and his grieving family was ordered to stay out in the waiting room while clinical triage staff tried to resuscitate him. Unfortunately, he could not be revived. Amohaere was called to intervene because the dead man's family was overly aggressive towards the doctors. 'As soon as I walked in the door, I could see the nurses on one side of the room and this whānau on the other. It was a stand-off. I was scared myself at the situation. Being a woman and not a fluent speaker of the reo was always prevalent in my mind when approaching male kaumātua like this.' The whānau rushed Amohaere when they heard her greet them with 'kia ora'. 'It was as if the air was cleared. All they wanted was one of their own who understood them and their needs, to know how he died and what would happen next.'

After speaking to the nurses, Amohaere asked if the whānau had a kaumātua or a spokesman, and together they were able to broker a meeting between the whole whānau, their spokesman and the resuscitation team. Amohaere says this was the first time that hospital staff had ever spoken directly to a family like this. There was tension in the air, but Amohaere's calming presence had prevented the police from being called. The sponteneity of the kuia's crying and the open show of emotion were foreign to the staff, who were distressed by the whole affair.

'I told the doctors to speak in simple language and to break down the jargon to make it easier for everyone to understand.' With all the facts and processes understood by the family, the aggression dissipated. Amohaere always maintained hospital staff needed to be cognisant of families' emotions, especially when their loved ones died in the wards. 'I don't think my colleagues realised the huge cultural pressure that went along with this role of bringing calm to these explosive situations. However, I was encouraged on this occasion when one of the kuia said to me, "Kei te pai girl!"'

It was further comforting when triage staff later called Amohaere into a debrief to thank her for her essential intervention in this situation. They recognised they had not known how to handle it. Perhaps the most telling factor was the fact that nurses witnessed immense change in so-called difficult patients and families once Amohaere's Māori process was effectively completed. This went a long way to confirming the need for her role in the hospital. 'We need this type of resource,' one of the senior doctors admitted.

*

The above scenario was one of many witnessed in the hospital where cultural sensitivity was lacking and silent offence was given to patients and their families. For the sake of communicating cultural awareness in the wards, a group was formed to discuss the relevant issues around this kaupapa and promote various ways to implement appropriate care. This led to the establishment of Te Roopu Kai Ārahi Ki Te Ora in 1988 to support the education of hospital staff on the Treaty of Waitangi, biculturalism and racism. As well as Amohaere in her role as parent liaison officer, others invited to rally together were Karena Way (anti-racism and Treaty of Waitangi education project manager), Caroline McKinney (chairperson of the Māori Nurses' Association), Doreen Arapai (a Niuean nurse), Debbie Sorrenson (a Tongan nurse in the hospital's crisis team), Ake Villiamu (Samoan senior nurse), Mahia Wallace (a kuia and founding member of the Māori Nurses' Association), Mata Forbes (charge nurse, Auckland Hospital), Mereana Solomon (in-service department) and others.

The call to support cultural awareness and safety in-house brought with it a number of tensions. Long-term Māori and Pacific hospital staff who well knew the cultural inadequacies of the current system and the lack of a voice in the organisation felt threatened or believed they should have been offered the parent liaison position. Senior nurses tried to have Amohaere and Karena Way removed from their positions. A fiery meeting of Māori staff was held where they were attacked. There was a sense that staff knew Māori needs had to be met, but additions such as the reo and the Treaty were not seen as essential components of care. There were personal and tribal jealousies at play as well. However, when supportive nurses and orderlies understood that Amohaere had a platform to speak at management level and the power to make changes, they realised they had an ally in her, not an enemy.

While Te Roopu Kai Ārahi Ki Te Ora had a multi-ethnic flavour, its aims were primarily to recognise and support tangata whenua.[14] It also encouraged and supported in-service departments in the education and delivery of appropriate Māori care as part of an overall outcome of good health for Māori and other groups.[15] The group met regularly and resolved to include all Māori staff at the hospital, at that time about 30 out of a total staff of 3000.

The hospital's mission statement included ensuring 'a commitment to Bicultural Health Service delivery on the basis of partnership in accordance with the Treaty of Waitangi and the provisions of care which is acceptable to all cultures'.[16]

The group proposed a new style of orientation programme (for new and established staff) that included sessions on the Treaty of Waitangi and bicultural awareness. Amohaere organised the first orientation day. Rooms were set aside and turned into a marae space with the first powhiri (welcome) and also the first-time involvement of kaumātua Doc Wikiriwhi of Ngāti Whātua as mana whenua in any hospital activity. The programme got off to a shaky start. There was strong resistance from hospital staff who didn't want a bar of it. Attendees either didn't arrive or were 'embarrassingly culturally insensitive'.[17] While the bicultural and Treaty workshops created a greater awareness of the growing need to work with Māori, for many hospital staff there was a sense that 'the Māori were taking over'. Most knew the Treaty had some significance to the nation but didn't see that biculturalism and Treaty education had any relevance to the world of clinical care.

There were cries that this Māori activism encroaching on hospital medical practice 'was utter lunacy'.[18] Doctors didn't see the point of taking working time out to be, as many saw it, abused and accused in these seminars. The extent of anti-Māori sentiment in the hospital was obvious. However, Mary Futter was totally committed. She publicly told staff if they didn't accept the Treaty education, perhaps they had better think of some other job.[19] This caused division, and those who couldn't take it did leave. She held firm in her belief that there was no disadvantage in taking this bicultural path.[20]

As management continued to push the requirement for staff to attend these orientation days, the climate of the hospital began to change. For example, there was loosening of restrictions on visiting hours, which meant parents now had greater access to the wards to be with their children.[21]

Te Roopu Kai Ārahi Ki Te Ora continued to support in-service departments in the education and delivery of Māori health, highlighting cultural awareness issues in the wards. It proposed taha Māori programmes, marae visits, a permanent base with resources, and funds to be made available for kaumātua volunteers and a co-ordinator at management level. The group sought an affirmative action employment policy, and institutional racism workshops were to be delivered to everyone on staff.[22]

As the idea of 'cultural safety' was so highly charged amongst non-Māori staff, it was decided to train people under the guise of 'bicultural best practice'. 'This language was not so confronting. We had to be wise and find words and terms that could fit easily into the common practice system,' Amohaere says.

Taking cultural safety from theory into practice was about identifying Māori concepts that could be aligned with the realities of the profession. It was more than simply addressing culture as art, carving and history or understanding marae protocols. It was about teaching Māori realities of hygiene, infection control, health and safety, and safe communication via professional examples of practice that exemplified and satisfied cultural difference. This often meant grouping Māori concepts under clinical labels in professional language for easy comprehension by nurses and doctors.

Amohaere's dream was to have medical professionals well versed in both clinical and Māori cultural competencies. Her first question was always, 'How do we walk alongside the professionals as Māori to ensure a better quality of wellness for Māori?'

The learning process in cultural awareness and culturally safe practice continued with in-service or mini seminars in the wards so that medical staff could quickly discuss any cultural issues that may have arisen on a day-to-day basis. Amohaere says that finding a clinical way to explain tikanga to medically minded people was paramount for easy understanding. Criticising hospital staff for common but inappropriate practices in the wards created resistance to the notion of cultural safety. However, when staff were told these cultural issues were primarily about hygiene, they took it on board. Simple issues such as using the same X-ray bolsters (padding) for both the patient's head and backside during an X-ray was culturally wrong for Māori, who regarded placing anything associated with the posterior and the head together as a breach of tapu.

Te Roopu Kai Ārahi Ki Te Ora bicultural action groups were created in the wards. Here, groups of Pākehā, Māori and Pacific Island nurses grappled with cultural values and how to apply them. Differentiating pillows designated for the head from those for the lower body took years to work out, yet it was as simple as using colour-coded pillowcases for the head, the posterior and other purposes. This was a solution one of the bicultural action groups came up with that revolutionised the way bedding was dealt with in hospitals. Before it became standard practice in the Auckland hospital system, though, the organisation needed to accept that this was even an issue. As well as being a good cross-infection control measure, it totally respected Māori cultural values.

Getting to this stage, where attitudes and practice could be tested and adjusted, was no easy task, but inroads were slowly being made through gentle persuasion and practical education.

SIX

Kāhui Kaumātua

When Amohaere first told her mother about her new job as parent liaison officer, Mary offered some cautionary advice. 'She said I must protect myself in the hospital setting because of the spiritual entities of sickness and death prevalent there. So I followed her advice, and I'd pray discreetly before entering and after leaving the hospital. It wasn't as if this was strange advice; the elders at home lived this way. Karakia was a normal part of life. The only thing was I was the one having to do the praying now.'

Amohaere realised she would have to step up into her own 'Māoriness' to carry out the mandate of her position. 'I thought I knew about things Māori, but I pretty quickly realised I didn't know much at all. Patients in the wards would speak Māori to me, and I couldn't answer them in the way that I should have. Issues to do with body parts and blood were continually raised, and I had minimal knowledge of tikanga on how to deal properly with those issues. I felt so ignorant and inadequate.'

Many times in that first year, she just wanted to step away altogether. 'My mother became my personal cultural advisor. She always had the right advice for me, and I'd do what she suggested was necessary. She was my rock.'

Expectations on Amohaere by staff and patients alike were high. She was the Māori liaison person therefore she must know everything about Māori issues and custom. This is an assumption commonly made by organisations about their Māori staff, but it simply isn't true. 'There were Māori specialists in tikanga, which I certainly was not. I needed a larger body of informed people who knew how to answer the hard cultural questions and discern what should happen when exceptional circumstances that needed a speedy cultural solution arose.'

As her responsibility and workload grew, Amohaere found herself walking between Princess Mary Hospital and the Auckland general hospital more regularly. She grappled with recurring incidents that needed deeper cultural understanding. Added to her own cultural limitations, there was the reality of being a young woman dealing with male Māori patients and whānau. Amohaere concluded that she needed the advice of elders knowledgable in Māori cultural aspects of health and wairuatanga (spirituality).

She approached her relative, kaumātua Toby Curtis, at Hato Petera College and a local kuia, Mahia Wallace, to advise her. Mahia was from Ngāti Tūhourangi, was living in Auckland and was an elder on the National Council of Māori Nurses. Having worked as a nurse in the wards, she had a great knowledge of the dilemmas Amohaere faced. Mahia graciously accompanied Amohaere on difficult occasions to meet with Māori families with children in the hospital. She was also instrumental in introducing Amohaere to tribal elders in the Auckland region to discuss the idea of gathering a team of kaumātua to advise the hospital on cultural matters.

One of the first elders Mahia introduced Amohaere to was the prominent Anglican minister, Canon John Thornton Rongotoa Tamahori. A man steeped in Māori thought and philosophy, he was also the past chaplain at Te Aute Māori Boy's College, Pukehou, Hawke's Bay, and, more recently, was lecturing on 'the Māori point of view' to priests training at St John's Theological College.[1] 'He was a large, gracious man, knowledgeable about my own whakapapa, who immediately saw the big picture. He advised kuia Mahia and I to gather a collective of kaumātua together and made a number of suggestions about who should be contacted.'

They visited other Auckland-based tribal elders like Doc Wikiriwhi, Ruby Gray, Danny Tumahai, John Turei, Rev. Eru Potaka Dewes, Rev. Hone Kaa, Brownie Williams and Te Pere Curtis, to name a few. Mahia called a hui with all the local tribal elders, chaired by Toby Curtis, where Ngāti Whatua were rightly recognised as the mana whenua. Because the city's hospital service catered to the needs of Māori from all tribes, it was felt a gathering of multi-tribal elders living in Auckland was right and proper.

More importantly, with the hospital standing within Ngāti Whātua territory, it was recognised that Ngāti Whātua must maintain its status as mana whenua within this forum. Historically speaking, Princess Mary Hospital and Auckland Hospital sat inside the original lands of central Auckland sold by Ngāti Whātua to the Crown. In 1840, 3000 acres were sold to the Crown for goods and cash worth £281 and another 13,000 acres from Waitemata to Manukau were sold by Ngāti Whātua in 1841 for £200 and goods.² Later still, portions of those purchased lands were resold to settlers at hugely marked-up prices. In the *Auckland Hospital Endowments* (WAI 261) Waitangi Tribunal claim interim report, proviso was made in the land transactions that 10 percent of subsequent land sales be returned to Ngāti Whātua in cash or services, namely for the founding of schools, the construction of hospitals and for the payment of medical attendance. There are contentions that 10 percent or the equivalent was never, in fact, given, and it was the subject of a commission of inquiry in 1927.³

The report highlights Governor Grey's reservation of 300 acres for the endowment of Auckland Hospital in 1850, taken from the 13,000 acres acquired from Ngāti Whātua, as an act of honouring his undertakings with Māori. However, that endowment passed, without payment, to the Auckland Area Health Board. There is a sense that the 'assurance of special hospital services for local Māori iwi was a part of the "price for Auckland"'.⁴

It took Mahia and Amohaere, out of working hours, a whole year of discussions with these elders, before the full potential of what they were forming and its function came to fruition. As Amohaere got to know the elders, she had an open door to contact them any time she needed. 'Usually if something arose in the wards, I'd consult with Ngāti Whātua first, where possible, then I'd seek another kaumātua view before moving forward on a decision.'

Many times she would visit the sick children's parents, accompanied by Mahia and Canon John, both of whom had a great understanding of protocol, an excellent command of Māori and English and a deep understanding of the dynamics and circumstances that had befallen Māori families.

All this played a major part in relationship-building between Princess Mary Hospital and the Māori community. The recognition of this essential relationship with tribal eldership was acknowledged publicly in October 1989 at an inaugural gathering in the Auckland Hospital grounds. This event formally established the elders as a Kāhui Kaumātua, a body of mana whenua and multi-tribal representatives of the Māori people of Auckland. More than one hundred people had gathered to formalise this agreement between Princess Mary Hospital management and the Kāhui Kaumātua. Canon Tamahori officiated. It was the first time any health organisation within the Auckland Area Health Board had formalised such a relationship. 'It was a rude awakening for the staff of the day who were finally to be privy to the presence of a full Māori contribution,' Amohaere reflects.

The Kāhui Kaumātua, created to provide cultural knowledge to the organisation for the needs of Māori people, had a great desire for the general upgrade of Māori health and eventually became part of a dual decision-making process alongside the hospital management team. Those elders who contributed to this council (1989–1994) were Canon John Tamahori, Mahia Wallace, Toby Curtis, Te Pere Curtis, John Turei, Bill Tāpuke, Dave Mackey, Doc Wikiriwhi, Danny Tumahai, Brownie Williams, Rangi Matehaere, Tamihana Thompson, Ngarau Tupai, Aronia Ahomiro, Mavis Rivers, Mita Makiha, Kito Pikahu, Amelia Oppenheim and Ihimaera Ihimaera. Others who supported the Kāhui Kaumātua and Te Whānau Atawhai were Rev. Eru Potaka Dewes, Rev. Hone Kaa, Haki Wihongi, Dave King, Ruby Gray, Celia Burkhart, Wally Te Ua and Mavis Tuoro.

*

The Kāhui Kaumātua were well aware their influence would be crucial in convincing Pākehā hospital managers and doctors of the need for working with them and Amohaere to create a more effective health service for Māori. They met once a month to talk about hospital issues brought up by Amohaere. 'These were the people who influenced me as I grew into this role. They were the experts in tikanga Māori, and I took my lead from them.' When she felt she was making no progress, the elders would always encourage her to stay where she was. They were forceful in their resolve that her presence in the hospital was much needed. They saw Amohaere's role as a forerunner for what was to come.

Meetings were held in the reo, and there were numerous debates on subjects such as tapu and noa in the context of clinical care. The belief in the idea of illness, or of making a person susceptible to unwellness, arising from an interference with personal tapu was still a prevalent view amongst Māori,[5] including this council of elders. This created a state of negative noa that needed rectifying through a process of restoring the patient's personal tapu and fostering a state of positive noa.[6]

Creating a meeting place for Māori whānau where common rituals could be attended to, or where on-site family accommodation could be found, was a pressing issue. The Whānau Room accommodation and later the Whānau Atawhai space on the top floor of the Starship Children's Hospital came about as a direct result of the elders' agitation. As mentioned earlier, many elders, including Brownie Williams, Aronia Ahomiro and Tamihana Thompson from Mataatua Marae in Māngere, volunteered their time to serve the families in these spaces. Their services were essential to the caring environment brought about by manaakitanga (respect and hospitality) and whanaungatanga (relationship).

Some of the reports to the Kāhui Kaumātua on hospital practice and aspects of Amohaere's role generated reactions of disgust, anger, silence and even denial or avoidance. This was certainly true of the reports Amohaere presented concerning the abuse of Māori children – something that was all too commonly seen in the hospital admissions. Of all the important topics to come across the elders' table for discussion, it was child abuse that was the most heartbreaking for them all. 'Hearing the reports and seeing the graphic images of abused Māori children, some of them close family members to the elders, was shocking for them to be confronted with.'

The kaumātua were shocked and frightened when she first began to share the reports along with the difficulties she had engaging with the Māori children's families. 'They were just not comfortable with what was occuring with our local whānau Māori. For years, many of our people had swept this subject under the carpet and kept silent,' she admits. The kaumātua were now exposed to this reality. It was a whole new world to many of them. Was this really happening in Māori homes? The elders debated long and hard about this subject and realised how difficult it was to create a safe environment of care for the children. The respect and honour that existed amongst Māori in an earlier generation was quickly being eroded. 'I explained to them how this issue was not going to disappear, but it would probably grow to a greater degree in the future.'

At the time, Amohaere was continually confronted with the state of sick and dying children, many of whom were abused. A high percentage were Māori, who very rarely had family accompany them into the hospitals. Statistics of the period showed that sudden infant death rates were alarmingly high among Māori infants under one year old. The rate was twice as high as for non-Māori and is largely attributed to cot death.[7] A number of reasons were proposed for this, including low birth weight (less than 2500 g), smoking in the baby's environment, sleeping position and socio-economic status.[8]

Child protection teams created within the hospital included Amohaere as the advocate for Māori families along with child health experts. The pediatric unit met regularly to present cases of the children whom they felt needed referral to the protection units for assessment. These assessments were carried out in conjunction with Social Welfare staff to gauge the level of safety needed for the child's future care. For the most part, these were children hospitalised for non-accidental injuries largely inflicted on them by adults. Many cases involved sexual abuse. One of the doctors sympathetic to a more cultural way of engagement and care for the children would show Amohaere the extent of injuries found on the children's bodies. Some of these children survived, some did not.

For Amohaere it was highly disturbing. She was no stranger to conflict in the home, 'But I tell you, I got a fright,' she says with conviction.

Because of continued suspicion by staff about Amohaere's role, she was initially denied full access to the files and the inner circle discussions about these children. Patient files were highly confidential, available only to the multidisciplinary staff involved in a patient's medical care. Because Amohaere was not a trained medical specialist or nurse, she says the medics were not sure why she would need access to the files or to make any comment on them. Her role was seen as simply one of social observation rather than one of clinical contribution.

However, Dr John Newman, head of the multidisciplinary (MD) team meetings at the time, realised that many of the files lacked information that could possibly help determine patient care and medication. Amohaere was able to bridge the gap with Māori families willing to sharing their secret concerns with her, and Dr Newman felt her perspective as the cultural voice of the patients was an integral one. Despite this, it would take some years before Amohaere was included in the MD meetings to comment or have access to patient files.

Sometimes, there was an immediate rapport between Amohaere and Māori whānau ushering their children into the hospital. 'Seeing a Māori face or hearing a familiar Māori greeting at the door was 75 percent of the healing of a patient and their family. They knew they were in an environment that might understand and not criticise them.'

Other times, having a Māori meet with the injured children and their whānau had no calming effect whatsoever. 'My role was to receive the Māori children at the door and then make contact with the families to enquire as to how the child had ended up this way. It was horrific. I couldn't understand why people would beat their children, sexually abuse them or burn them with cigarettes.' The police would inform the staff a Māori baby was being sent in to the hospital. The baby would be ushered to emergency care and a meeting would be organised with the assembled family. Usually the perpetrators would be present. 'I had to learn to control my emotions and be careful not to show my outrage. It wasn't about me – it was about these children.'

The level of violence inflicted on children was something she had never experienced before. 'I'd lie in bed at home and think about the ordeal these children had been through, and I realised how important this hospital position was to me and to the young patients' futures.' She later formed the idea that violence was multigenerational.

Making contact with patients' families was surprising to say the least. 'I'd connect with families either at a called meeting or in their own homes. The elders of the family would present themselves; these were people I had seen on the paepae (orators' bench) of the marae or who were in some kind of community leadership role. I could never understand how they could not know this kind of violence was going on in their own homes; how blind could they be? As the actions of these kaumātua and other family members was revealed, my respect for many elders diminished. I really had to control my own thoughts during family meetings.'

Often Amohaere had to step out of the meetings because she was either related to or knew the families involved or the perpetrator. This was a conflict of interest if she was called to make a judgement on these cases. 'I didn't want to meet the perpetrators really,' Amohaere admits.

Confidentiality was a paramount code of practice at all times. Any breach of it could be harmful for the patient or their family. There was a process in place if circumstances required the confidentiality of the patient to be breached. 'I had the highest respect for the specialist clinicians. They had integrity; their entire focus was for the children. They held no prejudice or hidden views towards the children or their families.' It was more of a struggle for Amohaere knowing full well who the perpetrators and their families were. The horrific incidents of abuse had a harrowing effect on her, and she sought private counselling for herself.

Phone calls to her mother were full of sobering advice. 'She would tell me it's not about me. She would encourage me. You can handle this, she'd say.'

Amohaere does not believe child abuse is particularly a Māori issue and neither did the pediatric staff. 'All cultures are guilty of violence, but at the time, a high percentage of child abuse cases entering the hospital were our own. The question was how do we break the stigma of this in the health sector?'

Amohaere conveyed to the Kāhui Kaumātua how families often had no information about how to handle the situation when they knew there was something wrong. Engaging with whānau was more about learning how to help them than judging them or creating a 'them' and 'us' scenario.

'I'd disclose enough information to the whānau to show them we were there to help them to walk together with us for the good of their child. This process could never be rushed,' she insists. Creating a rapport with many of these families who had longstanding violent backgrounds meant Amohaere having to dress, talk and act in a similar manner before an environment of trust could be created. 'We had to break the barrier of being accused of being "just like them" – judgmental white people. They had to get to know me as a person.'

The Kāhui Kaumātua advised Amohaere that wairuatanga (spirituality) and whakapapa (genealogy) were strong traditional concepts relevant to creating rapport with families. Families began to open up to Amohaere and the hospital, sometimes admitting they were wrong in their actions towards the child or children. On other occasions, the battered children's fathers or other men in the family would react to her visits with violent outbursts, and the police had to be called. Some families didn't want Amohaere involved. Often her links to wider family connections led to the families involved rejecting her presence in any meetings to safeguard their own confidentiality. They chose a Pākehā case worker.

Social workers, doctors and the police were all involved in the family plans for the protection, safety and care of the children. 'Our families were afraid of the power of social workers,' Amohaere says. The perpetrators were arrested or referred to particular social agencies, while many families could not resolve their issues or stay together any longer. 'Initially, I too was sceptical of the hospital system, but I realised I had to be in the system to bring about change. I was critical, but I learned to walk the road to change the small things.'

The Kāhui Kaumātua became a lot more involved in travelling with Amohaere to engage with the community on this issue. To their great credit, Rev. Hone Kaa and others associated with the Kāhui Kaumātua became champions for the safety and protection of childen in New Zealand. The issue of child abuse began to surface as a multigenerational problem, and as a response, Hone became more instrumental in supporting initiatives to advance Māori education and the protection of children and their families. From 2008, he served on the steering committee of Every Child Counts and was the Chair of Te Kāhui Mana Ririki Trust right up to his passing in 2012.

Karakia was always prevalent in the world of these kaumātua, the majority of whom were ministers of the cloth. Kaumātua were constantly called on to pray and deal with particular situations where a shift in the atmosphere of a space was needed, especially when a death had occurred. Amohaere's introduction to the mental health area at Auckland Hospital came when there was a suicide in Ward 10. Airini Tukerangi, the site nurse, walked her through the ward to the place where the suicide had occurred. The nurse wanted someone to come and bless the room and have someone explain from a Māori perspective why this needed to happen. 'You could feel death in the atmosphere. I rang up, and Doc Wikiriwhi came and performed the karakia for the ward and gave an explanation.'

Tribalism was still prevalent amongst the Māori families Amohaere met with at the hospital. Visiting families would ask 'Nō hea koe?' ('Where are you from?') as is common amongst Māori. However, when it was realised Amohaere wasn't from their tribal area, families would blatantly turn their backs on her. This behaviour appalled the Kāhui Kaumātua who couldn't believe this divisive attitude still existed, especially when one of their own was offering support in the alien environment of the hospital. When tribal issues arose in the wards with families, Kāhui Kaumātua elders of those particular iwi intervened to help.

*

Deep cultural issues like the removal of body parts, dealing with kēhua (ghosts) and wairua poke (haunting spirits), blessing rooms, understanding mate Māori (Māori sickness attributed to transgression of tapu), handling materoto (stillborn babies) or tūpāpaku (the body of a deceased), storing and returning the whenua (placenta) or pito (umbilical cord) to parents, family violence or the correct recital of karakia for whenua tohe (contested land), to mention just a few, were quickly brought to the elders' attention by Amohaere. Robust discussion ensued to ascertain the correct tikanga needed to be put in place in the hospital.

General talk amongst the elders about how to instigate cultural practice in the wards was all very well. But for Amohaere, nothing could ever be implemented unless policies were drawn up at board level and accepted as part of the hospital's strategy and values. The process of policy making went through a number of channels before it was tabled at board level.

One incident that forced a new policy to be written concerned the storage of a child's placenta. Amohaere was informed that nurses had saved a placenta for a family by storing it in a refrigerator where food was kept. After consulting with the kuia Mahia, Amohaere advised the nurses to find another fridge or, in the interim, to at least keep the placenta separated from food. Urban Māori families would often store their children's placentas in the food freezers out of necessity until it was convenient to traditionally bury them on their whānau lands, thereby reinforcing the relationship between the newborn and their traditional lands. However, by Māori cultural standards, the mixing of body parts with food was considered a defilement of tapu and unhygienic. 'Even if I didn't understand why it was wrong to mix the placenta with food, I knew by intuition what was wrong and what was tika (correct),' Amohaere says. She took the matter higher and was invited by the board to attend a meeting to explain the circumstances, to share the associated tikanga and to recommend change to ward practice. The subsequent policy outlined the correct storage procedure – placing the whenua and pito (umbilical cord) into a special container to be stored in a specific freezer that also would store other body parts – and educated staff about this topic.

As time went on, the hospital was increasingly open to hearing Amohaere's opinions, but the general manager explained how the organisation still needed written policies around these kaupapa before staff would follow in practice. Recording cultural rationale for tikanga and policies on paper was something the Kāhui Kaumātua had a deep aversion to. They didn't want their knowledge taken out of context then abused or stolen again. They were uncomfortable with publicly revealing their cultural practices in written form, especially inside a non-Māori institution. 'He momo ture Pākehā tēnā' (Just more white man's laws), the elders would say. 'Kei te tapu ērā kōrero' (Those things are sacred), they maintained.

Amohaere had to be firm with the elders and convey the message to them with the support of Canon Tamahori. 'Without the tikanga and mātauranga written on the page and contained within policy, nothing would happen, no change at all would occur.' With a gentle push and more involvement in the wards, the Kāhui Kaumātua conceded. This was a major decision for the elders and a major breakthrough for Amohaere.

There were still ethical issues to conquer in the area of policy making. One of the biggest hindrances was the ethical conflict between clinical practice and traditional rongoā practice, which clinicians commonly believed was unscientific and untested.

This was clearly illustrated in a case where doctors and Amohaere butted heads over the treatment of a Māori patient. He was being treated, with very little result, for a particularly aggressive cancer that had eaten through to the bone. The hospital staff wanted to continue clinical treatment, while the patient's family wanted to try traditional Māori rongoā. The clinicians would only agree to allowing the rongoā if they could control its administration, study the medicinal properties and closely monitor its progress. The forceful whānau were insistent that their intellectual property should remain secret and their sole property.

Amohaere became embroiled in the heated tension that grew between the two sides. With advice from the Kāhui Kaumātua, she persuaded the two factions to sit at the same table and converse. The doctors and the whānau tohunga met and shared their separate points of view. Always the diplomat, Amohaere made the point that they were all there for the patient, who, up to this point, had been left out of the discussion. He then made his voice heard.

He didn't want to stop the cancer treatment, but he would like to try the rongoā Māori medicinal poultice suggested by his family, under their terms. If it did not change his situation, he would return to just the clinical care. No one could argue the point.

The rongoā was applied to the man's body over a four-week period. When the poultice was removed both the tohunga and the doctors were amazed to see only a small scab over the hole in the flesh. For Amohaere it was a watershed moment. It was an illustration of the tense opposing attitudes expressed between clinical and traditional holistic experts, both suspicious of each other's practices. This could be seen as an example of the state of Māori and non-Māori realities when it came to health practice overall.

However, for the first time in Amohaere's career, medical specialists and Māori tohunga spoke in the same room, agreed and participated together, working alongside each other for the good of the patient. 'My wish was to find a way to bring the two realities together and create policy that recognised both the clinical and the holistic way for best practice and the wellness of our patients.'

*

The Kāhui Kaumātua elders' ready availability and attendance at meetings were purely on a voluntary basis. They were extremely busy people but understood the work at the hospitals was paramount. 'It became embarrassing after a while how much we had to rely on the elders' advice without any renumeration of any kind for them,' Amohaere remembers. 'There was no such thing as a koha (reciprocal gift) system in place to recognise their professional consultations.' Amohaere formally requested some kind of monetary payment as a koha to compensate for their time and knowledge. The accountants insisted this could not be done 'until one day one of the accountants informed me they had worked out a way for me to ask for a koha to be gifted to the elders. That was the first time the hospital had paid out for cultural advice. It was a small but great victory at the time.'

In saying that, none of the elders wanted to take money or any formal payment for their services. As far as they were concerned, they were there for the people. For Amohaere, this was a sign of their humility, but this attitude still did not cover the cost of their travel from their homes to the hospital or out into the communities. Eventually, remuneration in the form of a koha was accepted.

Changing the system often took its toll on Amohaere who found herself constantly at the coalface of the conflict of worldviews. 'I don't think I was fully prepared for the intensity of this role. It became hugely political, especially with the inclusion of the Kāhui Kaumātua in the mix. Pākehā challenged my every move, and the jealousy of my own colleagues was intense. Many times, I just didn't want to be there. I'd ring my mother so she could tell me to come home, but she and the other kuia encouraged me to stay where I was. They knew this was where I was meant to be.'

Canon Tamahori was always interested in Amohaere's progress. He recognised the heavy responsibility that went with the growing capacity of her position.

'Canon Tamahori would constantly enquire if I was okay personally. He was aware that being a woman in this environment meant I would come up against my fair share of racism and chauvinism from both Pākehā and Māori. He was always gracious enough to inform me to remember who I was and what I was there to do for the people. He was on call for me at any time and for any situation, to speak on my behalf whenever I felt I needed support. He was a wonderful man.'

Amohaere believes she was extremely privileged to sit amongst the elders at this revolutionary time.

'I knew my place as a woman, but the elders would always ask my opinion on specific subjects. In those days, I wasn't that confident in the company of Māori elders. They could be intimidating. Often, I'd ring my mother and she would tell me how to move amongst them. All their meetings were in the reo, and they all thought I could speak because they knew my whānau and had watched my son Pouroto's (Nicholas's) progress in the Māori world. But I certainly wasn't of the same calibre as any of my own whānau. I did not want to ride on their coat-tails either. I wanted to be me.'

Canon Tamahori, Mahia Wallace, Te Pere Curtis and Toby Curtis were her closest confidants, and they walked alongside her to advocate in many situations. 'Without the Kāhui Kaumātua I would have been lost in this system, having to deal with situations like blessing rooms or finding afterbirths in hospital fridges. These were often roles that traditionally men carried out. They were the ones experienced in how to deal culturally with these issues.'

Kuia Mahia was especially sympathetic, knowing some of the terrible situations Amohaere faced on a regular basis. When they met to debrief, the kuia would always ask, 'Who died today, dear?' It was with her that Amohaere was able to speak openly about her frustrations, thoughts and emotions and to unwind.

One thing that bothered both Amohaere and the Kāhui Kaumātua was the lack of acceptance of the Māori language, or any language other than English, as an essential element of health care. Negative attitudes towards the correct pronunciation of Māori words were part of a rigid Pākehā-dominated monolingual world that had deep roots within the institution. 'Frustrated and with my back against the wall, it was either fight or flight.'

Fed up with this disrespectful environment, it all got too much for Amohaere (who at that time was known as Judith). She remembers bursting into her colleague Karena Way's office one day, clearly frustrated and distressed by this continuous disrespect, and announcing, 'That's it! That's it! From now on, I will be called Amohaere.' From that day, staff had to get their tongues around her Māori name. Although she had taken a stand, this wasn't a spur-of-the-moment decision but one she'd had to seek advice from whānau about. She had returned to Te Teko to ask her mother and other kuia if she could take on the name Amohaere, her grandmother's name, as her own. The elders agreed unequivocally. 'Kei te pai' (It is good with us), they said.

So as both a mark of respect for her grandmother and as a proactive step to value the reo in the workplace, she was now answerable to only one name. Amohaere was reclaiming her Māori identity.

This situation applied to other cultures as well. During a regular meeting with multicultural staff in the hospital, the issue of language was raised. 'We tried to make connection with the patients of other nations to open the doors of their world to the hospital. Most of the perceptions we as Māori had about hospitals, these other peoples shared with us.'

'I remember a Samoan family sitting in with their child, but no one had the language skills to communicate with them at the time. When I walked into the ward, I greeted them in Samoan after first learning their greeting from a Samoan nurse. The family automatically thought I was Samoan and launched into a long conversation with me in their language – a conversation I could not continue,' she admits. 'I didn't have permission to speak Samoan and raised false expectations with this family who were disappointed I couldn't converse with them.' When Ake Viliamu Malu, a Samoan nurse on duty, met the family, she was able to speak with them. She apologised on Amohaere's behalf for raising their hopes, asked Amohaere to call her if a similar situation arose again and told Amohaere in no uncertain terms that she needed to know her place.

Out of that situation, Amohaere was introduced to the Pacific community who were excited to meet a cross-cultural liaison worker from the hospital to share their worries about the relationship between their own customary values and the hospital system. 'They were gracious people who knew that as tangata whenua Māori needed to lead the charge on the political front to change the system. They would then follow in our footsteps.'

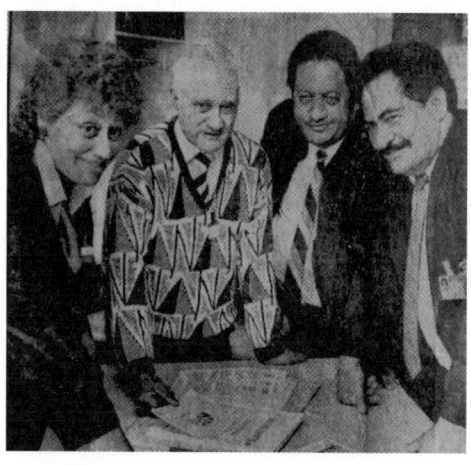

Amohaere with Kāhui Kaumātua members Te Pere Curtis, Brownie Williams and Aronia Ahomiro.
COURTESY OF TE WHĀNAU ATAWHAI ARCHIVES

SEVEN

The Challenge for Dignity

The notion of human dignity as 'the state or quality of being worthy of honour or respect'[1] is a core aspect of engagement between health professionals and the public. Dignity as a fundamental human right is all about being treated and regarded as important and valuable in relation to others. Its meaning is varied amongst the diversity of humanity. One Māori language translation of the concept of dignity is 'whakarangatira' – to revere, venerate, honour.[2] This is a concept intertwined with the personal mana of an individual and strongly related to 'the importance of respecting individuals and their right to dignity'.[3]

Māori were often suspicious of not being treated with respect and dignity, especially when anaesthetised in the operating theatre.[4] Not knowing how their bodies would be regarded or treated by strangers in the theatre was, and still is, a big concern. Treating a patient with privacy, modesty, respect and courtesy maintains dignity and should be the first consideration of health professionals in their management of patients.

Understanding the dignity of people and people groups is a whole separate dimension that can only be understood through the interface between self and the culture of peoples of difference. Cultural safety was designed to bring into nursing education and practice the respect for difference and the recognition of how one's own learned personal prejudices can influence how a person in a caring role may act towards those of different ethnicity and cultures.

As Amohaere walked the wards, she intuitively recognised practices that were contrary to dignity as expressed in the common Māori world that she knew. She witnessed this in attitudes towards both living and deceased patients.

A strong aspect of Māori cultural dignity is applied to death and dying, which is a very visible part of any hospital environment.

The lack of dignity Amohaere often witnessed towards the dead and the transgressions of tapu associated with the removal and disposal of bodies and body parts were of major concern. The subject of body parts had been highlighted in her own adult life when her mother brought the issue up after Amohaere had her first hip replacement operation. After a very bad fall in 1985, Amohaere was referred to a specialist orthopedic surgeon. An old sports injury from her pre-teen years had developed into arthritis and needed urgent attention. It appeared she needed a full hip replacement. Interestingly enough, when Amohaere was eleven, she'd fallen during a netball game, injuring her hip, and was in hospital for seven months. During this time, her father arrived to visit her on his motorbike, bringing Aunty Maraea Hunia from Te Teko, a woman with healing hands. She massaged the injury while muttering words under her breath. When the specialists of that time X-rayed Amohaere just prior to operating, they found the bones had miraculously healed and cancelled the operation. It was only in recent years that she realised her aunt Maraea had the gift of healing, specifically for bones. This was something the community was always silent and discreet about, but everyone knew who the specialised healers were when needed.

The full hip operation was carried out at the Mater Private Hospital in Remuera, once run by the Sisters of Mercy. At this time in her life, Amohaere had never had cause to mix in a white middle-class environment. 'It was a frightening experience being wheeled into a sterile theatre in a totally unfamiliar place with old Pākehā people who were about to tinker with my body. I couldn't fathom it really.'

The operation lasted five hours, and she was left to recouperate in the ward alone for two weeks with no communication, no explanation of what had occurred in surgery and no visitors. When she finally spoke with her mother about the operation, the only thing her mother was concerned about was where her orignal hip bones had gone. 'I didn't have any idea what she was talking about and why she would even want to know where my removed bones had gone.' As was the custom of the people, Amohaere's mother wanted those parts of her daughter's body that had been removed to be returned home and buried in the urupā. The completeness of a person's body was important. 'But my mother somehow knew she would never get the body parts back.'

Reminiscing about this simple procedure, Amohaere realised the Mater had never asked for her personal consent to dispose of her body parts and never enquired whether she wanted the remains returned to her. This was the way of New Zealand hospitals. It seemed to be the common perception that patients were either not interested in the return of body parts or doctors saw no need to offer them back to their patients.

When Amohaere took up the parent liaison position, she made sure pediatric doctors at management level understood the need for consent policies to ensure that body parts removed during surgery or post-mortem were able to be offered back to family members to dispose of in the appropriate cultural manner. To have this concept valued or even ratified was going to take time.

Amohaere also knew Māori were concerned about being accorded proper respect and dignity in the operating theatre. Many had spiritual concerns about the status of their wairua (spirit) during the anaesthesia process and how their mauri (life source) was being protected and preserved. Not surprisingly, there was resistance to her monitoring the behaviour of theatre staff. There was a sense that she had no right to be in the theatre and no need to add a Māori perspective to this arena, which was ususally reserved exclusively for clinicians. She had to force her way in to observe.

Through her own cultural lens, Amohaere saw that respect for the tapu and mana of an individual was lacking. Patients were left naked in front of strangers, their bodies disrespectfully prodded and the removed body parts treated without manaaki and respect. After an operation, patients were totally unaware of what had occurred while they were under anaesthetic.

Amohaere wanted her own people, or anybody for that matter, to be treated with dignity and respect. 'Once doctors and staff began to trust my presence and my worth in the wards, I was allowed access to the operating theatre. I always felt initially that once patients were anaesthetised, staff felt they had a licence to comment on, mock or treat a person's body how they liked. There was a lack of regard for the spiritual. Was this Pākehā culture at play? If a patient died, there was often an attitude amongst the staff that the deceased was now just a piece of meat. I felt the offence on behalf of the patients, and I'd express it openly. What I'd say would get around the hospital like quick-fire, and I'd be confronted by staff. My reply was always, "That could be you lying on that bed one day."'

In discussions with the Kāhui Kaumātua, it was made clear that whānau should be given the option to have karakia before an operation to ensure that the patient's spiritual, as well as physical, welfare was being properly looked after. In addition, pre-operative discussions should ascertain what other concerns the whānau and patient had and how they could best be addressed. As always, frank, open conversations ahead of time can, when sensitively handled, prevent untoward situations from developing.

*

Death can become so present in the day-to-day affairs of the hospital staff that they can become desensitised to it and even more so to the post-death processes. Death, imminent death and the removal and disposal of body parts in the hospital setting were all subjects for major discussions in the Kāhui Kaumātua camp.

Death and dying are so deeply imbued with cultural significance that whānau members from all over the country will usually hurry to visit or stay with a dying patient. This was often in conflict with hospital procedure.

The dignity of people in life and death was integral to the dialogue on tapu and mana – sacredness, separation and authority – of a patient and their family. The elders agreed that the manifestation of dignity should be expressed through the respectful conduct of staff for both the living and the dead in the hospital. Unfortunately, this was not the case in this era.

When children passed away in the wards, parents left standing at their child's bedside often did not know what would happen next. Normal practice was that the parents were asked to release the child's body to be taken to the mortuary for an autopsy, if required, and for it to be held there until funeral services could be organised. Amohaere remembers there was little communication between staff and families, so she would intervene and tell the whānau what processes needed to be followed for their loved one. 'I had to ask the families what they wanted for their child, but most did not know. More often than not, they were scared of death, so I'd have to suggest a way to move forward. This at least offered them some comfort, and they knew exactly what was happening with their child. Being with the family was a priority for me when a death occurred – even to the point of ensuring I would accompany their child to the mortuary and stay with the tūpāpaku, sometimes overnight, until whānau were ready to receive their child back again.'

Having no fear of death herself and having learned to dress the dead as a youngster, Amohaere encouraged the nurses to offer the parents the right to dress their own children to keep that connection between them before they were removed to the mortuary or funeral processes got underway. On other occasions, Amohaere would herself help prepare the deceased properly for the family to receive their loved one.

Post-mortems are often legally required, and there is no doubt this process disfigures the body. It also causes delays, which may impose additional burdens on the bereaved family who are, by custom, obliged to feed and house waiting mourners. Some Māori believe the spirit of the deceased is left alone with the body while it lies in the morgue. Also, some believe that the body requires all of its parts for the spiritual journey after death.[5]

On one occasion, after spending a lengthy time by a particular child's side prior to her passing, the family asked if they could accompany the child to the mortuary so that she would not be alone. Amohaere told them that this would not be allowed but volunteered to accompany the child to the mortuary and help to have her body released to them as soon as possible. Out of aroha (love) for the whānau, Amohaere even offered to bring the dead child north to their marae.

On that occasion, it was 3 p.m. by the time Amohaere, accompanied by health worker Manurere Dimitrof and Kaumātua Te Pere Curtis, arrived at the mortuary with the child's body. That was the usual time the pathologist finished work for the day, but because Amohaere had a good relationship with him, he agreed to her request to prepare the baby for the undertakers the family had already organised. Gaining this agreement took some doing. It was only after Amohaere had threatened to stay in the mortuary overnight with the child that the pathologist prepared the child and graciously gave permission for Amohaere and Te Pere to later uplift her.

'This was the first time he had ever been asked to prepare a tūpāpaku outside of hours for a cultural reason,' Amohaere recalls. 'I didn't think we were breaking any rules at the time; we just did what came culturally naturally to us.'

Amohaere and Te Pere then travelled during the middle of the night to carry the baby home. As a member of Te Arawa tribe, Te Pere was not comfortable taking the baby onto the marae at that time of the night. However, Amohaere already had instructions from the family elders to bring the child directly onto the marae no matter what time of night they arrived. Te Pere was indignant about this, but after he'd talked to one of the family elders about Ngā Puhi protocol (which allows people to come onto the marae at night), he was satisfied. Carrying the child onto the marae was acknowledged with great gratitude by the families, who recognised Te Pere's great mana as a kaumātua for accompanying their mokopuna home in this manner. 'I forced the issue without thinking it through,' Amohaere admits. 'Rather than wait for a process to be put into place, I wanted the family to have their child in their embrace as soon as possible.'

*

'There was often little respect for the dead in the mortuary,' Amohaere reflects. 'Bodies were thrown onto metal gurneys or benches with little dignity. They were just considered lifeless nobodies when they were, after all, someone's loved one.'

The mortuary is basically a freezer where tūpāpaku are stored until the pathologist can dissect and examine the body to ascertain the cause of death before handing it over to the undertakers. In certain cases, research is carried out to aid developments in finding cures for particular diseases.

Amohaere maintains that Māori have always had an aversion to the hidden procedures of the mortuary. There was concern that their loved ones' bodies were being tampered with or desecrated in some way and their body parts, no matter how minute the extraction might be, taken without consent for research purposes. Because of this, family members were cautious about allowing their deceased loved ones to be taken to the mortuary unaccompanied. Further to this, families would accuse the hospital of retaining their dead children's body parts after the bodies had been uplifted. They would demand the immediate return of these parts.

'One day, Te Pere Curtis arrived in my office ranting and raving on behalf of a family in mourning over one of their deceased loved ones, who, they believed, did not have their body parts returned by the hospital,' Amohaere recalls. He demanded their immediate return. Amohaere was keen to know how they had discerned this. Did the family do an in-depth examination of the tūpāpaku? How did they perceive this had occurred?

Te Pere was adamant the whānau were correct and demanded that she double-check with the doctors. In following up with the specialists, it was revealed the body part was still in the mortuary waiting to be tested. Somehow, the body had been released before the tests had been completed. In this case, it was a genuine mistake, and eventually the tūpāpaku was brought back to the mortuary where the organ was returned so the body could be buried in its entirety.

'I too held the same views concerning the mortuary without really understanding what goes on at an autopsy. It wasn't till I learned what the role of the pathologist was and observed dissection, examination and the tests carried out to ascertain the cause of death of a patient that I changed my mind,' Amohaere admits.

She and Te Pere were curious to understand and observe the mortuary process. Both were pleased to have their questions about the autopsies thoroughly answered. Body parts were examined for research purposes, and while the manipulation of the body during the process seemed disrespectful and undignified overall, after a lot of conversation and thought, both Amohaere and Te Pere came to the conclusion the procedure was both essential and unpreventable. 'When families request to be with their loved ones right through the whole pathology process, I say no these days. I say it would not be advisable. However, I was able to inform the families about the whole process, which effectively lifted any tension between the families and the hospital,' she says.

Another customary reason that the body is usually not left alone or unattended is to safeguard the tūpāpaku from being taken by others against the family's wishes. To do so is considered an unloving act. Additionally, it is believed by some that the spirit of the deceased wanders, and during the vital days of the spirit's movements, whānau should be present to mourn over and protect the wairua.[6] The practicality of carrying out this custom in the hospital was not necessarily viable. There were times in the ward where Māori people had passed away in the hospital, but circumstances didn't allow for large numbers of family to be present with their loved one.

Working with tūpāpaku from a cultural perspective and understanding the processes of the mortuary and funeral services became a serious topic of debate. The need for some tikanga around working with tūpāpaku became evident in teaching practices at the medical school. With more Māori students entering medical school, many were concerned about working with human cadavers as part of their training. Toby Curtis and others began to offer lectures on cultural competency and culturally appropriate practice as part of the teaching curriculum at Auckland Medical School. Kāhui Kaumātua elder Hone Kaa instituted tikanga theory and practice for the Māori students where karakia were recited prior to working with the cadavers and again at the end of the last teaching session with them. This was requested by the Māori students themselves when they were faced with a situation they felt needed Māori tikanga to create an atmosphere of cultural safety for them.

Critical to ensuring dignity is the concept of whanaungatanga. Kin connections to whānau, hapū and iwi are maintained and also extended to develop a sense of relationship between non-kin staff, patients and whānau and to create a cohesive caring family environment. This was well needed in a system that took a dim view of relating to patients and families in any personal way.

'I was committed to the patients and their families – so much so I'd go to their homes to attend the tangi of children that had passed away in the ward.

For a short time, I had become part of those children's lives, and I felt it was my duty as a Māori to show honour and whanaungatanga. Otherwise, we were just going back to old-time thinking and maintaining unwellness all over again,' Amohaere says.

On one occasion, when a young Pākehā girl passed away in the children's ward, Amohaere stepped in to cater for the needs of the distraught family. This included calling in a minister to come and pray with the family and lay the girl's spirit to rest. 'These small acts of aroha and respect are not solely Māori-related values.' When Amohaere came by the ward again, the girl's father was waiting in the corridor for her. He embraced her with a strong hug of gratitude for this small gesture of respect for his daughter. 'When you are part of something like that, you become emotionally connected, and we needed to learn to respond accordingly for the sake of these families.'

Because these whanaungatanga ideals were instilled in Amohaere during her upbringing, she was always conscious of the duties required at the death of a patient and mindful of the feelings of the family thrust into mourning. Working in the hospital, she was always deeply concerned as to whether the correct cultural procedures she was used to would be carried out for the tūpāpaku and the mourning family. Often, while the tūpāpaku was in the ward or held in the mortuary, Amohaere would keep the deceased company or even sleep alongside the body to ensure he or she was never left alone. Amohaere saw it as her duty to keep the Māori deceased company, even in the mortuary, until the whānau could come and claim their loved ones.

In critical care, there were rooms set aside where those who were on the edge of death would be taken and where limited numbers of family could spend the last moments privately with their loved ones. These were tagged 'the dying place'.

'When our people passed away in the hospitals, there was usually no karakia, no blessings, no emotion and no place for tangihanga.' 'The dying place' was less than adequate in Amohaere's view. A lot of people died in the hospital alone. These patients were often scared of dying alone, but attempts to find their families were often futile.

'One old kaumātua was dying in hospital but never had any whānau visit. I made him as comfortable as possible, but he eventually died alone. It wasn't till afterwards we found he was from Te Puna and was closely related to my father. I wept when I realised this too late, but we accompanied him home to his people. On arrival amongst his own tribe, the people thought he had died a long time before because no one had maintained a relationship with him for years.'

Because this was such a common state for many Māori, Amohaere and many others pondered how it got to this state. Where did the sense of whānau go? 'What I wanted was the maintenance and retention of whanaungatanga and dignity to operate for the good of everybody in the hospital, whether living or passed away. We were a multicultural hospital, and we, as staff, needed to take that into account.'

*

Terminally ill patients with highly contagious diseases were often hidden away in wards where visitors were restricted and patients were left to their fate in a very lonely state. In the 1980s, this was true of hospitalised patients with acquired immune deficiency syndrome (AIDS) – at that time a death sentence. After being called into one of the wards at Auckland Hospital, Amohaere chanced upon a number of Māori patients in a secluded ward. She was told they were AIDS patients isolated due to their condition and was denied access to that space. There was still suspicion amongst staff about her cultural liaison role, and it was going to take time for people to learn to trust her.

After a lengthy discussion with nurses on this particular ward, she was reluctantly allowed to see the Māori patients. Due to the nature of this illness, the names of patients presented on the boards were fictitious, and a big sign on the door read 'No Visitors'.

'Māori patients here needed manaaki and awhi no matter what state they were in. I'd go in to meet these men and hug them despite their contagious condition. They were so lonely, and they'd cry. It choked me up and changed me a lot. To see another Māori face was a relief to them, and their stories were so sad. There were no visitors, no family, absolutely nobody to comfort them; they had been rejected by the world.'

Many of these men died alone in a foetal position. Their bodies would be taken to the mortuary, blessed by the hospital chaplains, prepared in a specific manner due to the disease, then buried in a pauper's grave, unknown to anybody.

Overwhelmed by the men's suffering, Amohaere organised one of her own family members to come and keep them company. 'He understood the plight of these men and came at my request to sit and talk, to cry and comfort these dying patients.'

Comforting those in hospital with a terminal illness despite their colour, creed, or sexual orientation was part of Amohaere's Māori ethos to intentionally provide a measure of dignity and wellness from a cultural perspective.

Amohaere realised too that she knew many of their families. She decided to make contact with the families, most of whom had actually abandoned the men because of their sexual orientation. They had lost all contact with their sons or brothers and had been separated for many years. Her role encompassed contacting the families and informing them of the present state of their sons. Some never came. For others, it wasn't hard to persuade them to come and visit their own whānau again before they passed away, not afterwards.

Amohaere remembers telling one patient, to his total disbelief, that his family was coming to visit him soon. 'Really?' was his reply. 'I waited at the hospital entrance for this family to arrive, and when they came through the doors, I informed them of the situation then ushered them into the ward to visit their son and brother. There were many tears, lots of emotion and a great deal of reconciliation.'

It was heartbreaking for her to see families who were unable to touch their loved ones because of the infectious nature of the illness. 'It was an eye-opener for me. I learned to get over my own prejudices towards AIDS victims. Whanaungatanga and manaakitanga had to bypass all of that.'

Sharing with the Kāhui Kaumātua about the nature of caring for AIDS patients in the wards became a topic of long conversation with regard to the tapu of bed linen, cleanliness, blessings of rooms and tangihanga practice. Because of the life-threatening nature of the disease, this had ramifications not only for hospital hygiene and marae mourning processes but also for burial. Open coffins on the marae were prohibited in these cases, and tūpāpaku had to be wrapped in special shrouds.

These issues around dying and death within the hospital, revealing what occurred in the wards on a daily basis, brought to light many situations that were dealt with contrary to Māori customary practice. There was a great deal of robust debate after Amohaere's reports to the Kāhui Kaumātua about how to find tikanga-based solutions. This process also became a safeguard for Amohaere and the growing team of Māori staff entering the hospital system.

EIGHT

Te Whānau Atawhai

The Kāhui Kaumātua had a vision of an in-house Māori service for Auckland hospitals. Their strong desire emerged on the heels of a growing national cultural consciousness and a great deal of political agitation, particularly in the 1980s, for greater recognition by the State of Māori language, tikanga and self-determination.

A more bicultural approach to health governance and practice was raised by Māori who wanted to be involved in the planning and implementation of health services more suited to their people. Māori sought a system that would promote the positive acknowledgement of cultural values and practices.

Leading up to the late 1980s, Māori cultural models of care had emerged. The concept of health as an interaction between wairua, hinengaro, tinana and whānau was first presented during a training session for field workers in the Māori Women's Welfare League project, Rapuora, in 1982.[1] It was later created into a four-part framework known as Te Whare Tapa Whā (The Four-Sided House) by Dr Mason Durie, who introduced it as a health model in 1983 at a Young Māori Conference at Te Wānanga o Raukawa.[2]

Māori believed relationships with the medical profession had become strained because they felt the delivery of service was more narrowly focused on a colonial view of physical clinical care. There was no consideration of the spiritual aspects of the whole person. Māori embraced the Whare Tapa Whā model of health care and other alternative systems such as Te Wheke (The Octopus) and Ngā Pou Mana (The Pillars) in a move to reclaim a more positive and cultural shaping of health services.[3]

In 1983 at Tokanui Psychiatric Hospital, Te Roopu Awhina o Tokanui, a group of Māori health professionals, created the Whaiora Unit. Here, Māori values were actively promoted and introduced into health services in the belief that outcomes would be improved if the delivery was more relevant to the consumers.[4] The nine-part framework the Whaiora Unit promoted consisted of taha wairua (spirituality), taha whānau (family), taha hinengaro (mind), taha tinana (body), taha whenua (environment), taha tikanga (compliance), Māoritanga (old world), Pākehātanga (new world) and taha tangata (self).[5]

A similar promotion of Māori values was instigated at the Oakley Psychiatric Hospital in Auckland. By 1987, Oakley had closed and the M3 and M7 wards became part of Carrington Hospital. M7 (Male 7) was refurbished and became a special ward that was renamed Whare Paia.[6] This Māori Mental Health Unit managed by Titewhai Harawira advocated treating Māori patients in a culturally sensitive manner, but it soon ran into major difficulties, which created an unfortunate backlash towards Māori, particularly in the attitudes of non-Māori staff at other hospitals.

While iwi involvement in health policy and programmes was not extensive prior to 1984, there were a few health clinic initiatives in operation at the time. These included the Maaka Health Clinic in Ruatoki and a Tainui clinic on Waahi Marae. Whaioranga Trust in Tauranga was delivering health promotional programmes from Te Whetu Marae, and Ngati Raukawa had created a health committee.[7]

In 1984 Te Hui Whakaoranga (the Māori Health Planning Workshop) was a landmark gathering that sought to incorporate Māori health perspectives into the delivery of health programmes, increase the professional Māori health workforce, and develop Māori health organisations for Māori by Māori.[8] Held at Hoani Waititi Marae in Auckland, it was an initiative run by doctors Paratene Ngata, Eru Pomare, Lorna Dyall, George Salmond and Mason Durie.

In 1987, Irihapeti Ramsden, a Māori nurse advisor, educationalist and pioneer of culturally safe nursing practice, was seconded to the Department of Education as part of its commitment to biculturalism. Her task was to assist in the development of 'cultural safety' guidelines for the curriculum in safe nursing and midwifery education.

Cultural safety was a hugely controversial issue that was misinterpreted as an ethnic issue rather than being understood within its true concept, which was 'to improve the health status of all New Zealanders through the relationship between Māori and the Crown based on the Treaty of Waitangi'. Its emphasis, however, was on race relations and the relationship between nurses, midwives and their health service consumers/clients, who came from different cultural backgrounds. It wasn't until 1991, however, that the Nursing Council of New Zealand made cultural safety a requirement in the state examinations for nurses and midwives. The council commissioned the writing of guidelines to assist in the implementation of cultural safety into nursing and midwifery education. These guidelines known as the *Kawa Whakaruruhau* were written by Irihapeti Ramsden and finally adopted by the Nursing Council in 1992.[9]

The concept was born amidst controversial public debate with resistance fuelled by the media. 'Cultural safety' was associated with 'political correctness' and 'social engineering', raising doubts in the minds of the public and politicians about the quality of nursing education.[10] The word 'cultural' brought about confusion as people began to misinterpret it in this context as meaning 'ethnicity' or, more to the point, 'Māori'.

Cultural awareness and cultural sensitivity are both about having knowledge of an ethnic culture and ethnic diversity, whereas cultural safety was more about addressing the painful issue of race relations and racism.[11] It was never about learning Māori custom. Its original premise of improving the health status of all New Zealanders based on Treaty relationships has been further defined to 'include an emphasis on the relationship between nurses, midwives and health service consumers who differ to them by; age or generation; gender; sexual orientation; socioeconomic status; ethnic origin; religious and spiritual belief; disability'.[12]

Historically, generations of graduating nurses had sworn to the now obsolete Florence Nightingale oath to nurse people 'regardless' of colour or creed. However, in the modern era, recognising difference and the unconscious negative attitudes of nurses towards those differences became imperative for high quality care. Cultural safety required nurses to care for people 'regardful' of those things that make them unique.[13]

It is clear Māori were seeking a new and more positive paradigm for health services, incorporating not only western clinical care but also integrating Māori concepts of care and wellbeing. The relevance of culture to health professionals had become a significant issue by 1985, and Mason Durie cites the National Conference on the Role of the Doctor in New Zealand as recognising culture as a basis for health.[14]

Not everyone was impressed by these moves to return to a seemingly romantic vision of the past, with spiritual concepts that could not be measured or applied in practice.[15] However, the New Zealand Board of Health's 1988 recommendations for a national health policy advocated five principles:

holism, empowerment, social and cultural determination, equity of access and devolution, and equitable and effective resource use. These were all ideas borrowed from Māori views and writings.[16]

*

These events provided the ideological building blocks for change within the hospital system in which Amohaere was now employed. A philosophical shift in attitude was one thing, but identifying and recognising the need for a shift in practical terms in the wards was a totally separate ball game.

Amohaere remembers the kuia Pia Makiha, a former health worker prior to 1980, who would arrive at the hospital to visit Amohaere regularly to share her experiences of rampant unsafe systemic practices and her thoughts for the future. The time to bring some changes to that system was well overdue, but convincing the right people at the right level, with good cultural rationale and persuasive arguments, to make changes to policy and practice was a huge challenge.

It was no mean feat for a small contingent of agitators for culturally sound hospital practices to win the hearts of the decision makers inside the system. In saying that, some hospital managers had begun to realise the value of the Māori component to health – both to the community and to the hospital.

With some persuasion, Dr John Newman, the then head of the children's hospital, recognised the growing need for this kind of service. He approached Amohaere, with the support of the Kāhui Kaumātua, to take on a new role as Manager Māori Health. It was to be a salaried position with an operational budget and, more importantly, a greater authority to speak at board level. 'I wasn't looking for a leadership role at the time,' Amohaere insists, 'but I was pleased Māori leadership was now being accepted.'

With Dr Newman's influence and with other Pākehā colleagues as allies, the hospital had taken ownership of its responsibility towards a bicultural response. With any new move, there needs to be a face and a voice for the cause, and Amohaere was persuaded by the Kāhui Kaumātua to move forward and accept this opportunity.

The combination of sweeping changes in government policy and plans underway to build a new children's hospital provided a perfect prospect for the vision of a Māori family support unit to be realised. Dr Newman, as general manager of the new hospital-to-be, invited Amohaere to an executive meeting to discuss the options for utilisation of the projected seventh level.[17] Amohaere was now the voice of that vision. It was she who would have to face the executive decision makers. 'I was hesitant and terrified about attending this meeting. This was more to do with my lack of confidence to stand in front of professionals than anything else. But I was obliged to front up.'

Walking into the room of thirty or so medical executives and doctors was certainly intimidating. Despite her new title, Amohaere considered herself more a roots-level person than a high-flyer executive type. The Chief Executive of hospital management, Dave King, confronted Dr Newman as to who the new person in the room was. Dr Newman promptly introduced Amohaere, who was then given the floor to explain why it was fundamental that a Māori family unit be established within the new hospital structure. Amohaere was put on the spot to speak about the issues families were currently facing when visiting their children without accommodation being available. 'Families need space,' Amohaere maintained.

Some of those present were very vocal in their belief that there was no need for such a unit. They were sceptical of backing something that had never been tried or tested before. 'I quickly realised if you want to have an influence at management level you had to attend every meeting to be able to gently contribute to plans.' After lengthy debate and deliberation, the management committee made a decision.

Later, Dr Newman came down to see her. 'We've got it, Amohaere!' he exclaimed ecstatically. The board had accepted her concept as having a definable and necessary role in the future of client health initiatives, and space was allocated on the seventh floor for the use of the unit.[18]

'As I am a reserved person, I didn't think of the enormity of this decision. It took a while for what actually happened to sink in,' Amohaere reflects.

From being initially challenged by biculturalism and Treaty awareness, antagonist Dr Newman was to become Amohaere's greatest advocate in supporting a combined approach to care. In the early 1980s, he was part of a rheumatic fever advisory group in association with the Māori Women's Welfare League under Dame Whina Cooper. Attending two national Māori health hui in Rotorua and the Hui Whakaoranga at Hoani Waititi Marae 1984, he realised that the clinical approach was not sufficient to restore full health to Māori. Attending these hui were uncomfortable for him.[19] The high rate of rheumatic fever amongst Māori was considered by some quarters to be a 'Māori problem' governed by hereditary Māori genes. Dame Whina Cooper vehemently refuted this, claiming it was more to do with social and economic circumstances. 'It's the water,' she proclaimed. Dr Newman had his eyes opened to this, especially after becoming familiar with an article by Dr Rina Moore published in *Te Ao Hou* in 1960. She reiterated Dame Whina's position on social disparity, commenting that TB and rheumatic fever were ten times more prevalent in Māori than Europeans.[20] She identified poor housing, overcrowding, poor water supply, bad sanitation, the reluctance to allow doctors to come to the sub-standard housing, and the reluctance of women to visit male doctors as contributors to cross-infection and sub-standard health.[21]

Professionals like Dr Newman and hospitals in general had never considered the cultural or social circumstances of the people. In reality, they were only treating the symptoms of Māori unwellness. A new approach to health was needed; the big question in Dr Newman's and Amohaere's minds was how. Amohaere believed that becoming more whānau or family-centred was one vital step towards a new approach to care.

'In my view, the clinical world had lost its need to love the kids and their families.' Amohaere was the first to open Dr Newman's eyes to how hard it was for Māori to fit in with the medical system of the day. The trick was how they could work together.

'We all believed the Treaty had a place in New Zealand and we were obligated to look after Māori, but on our terms', Dr Newman says. 'I realised we could not get clinical practice where we wanted it to be without interacting with Māori. It was exciting times where opportunities to find solutions for Māori client disparity could be rectified.'[22]

When Dr Newman shared his vision for the new children's hospital (Starship) he outlined his belief in the hospital becoming a bicultural unit. He considered it to be the institution's obligation to adhere to the principles of the Treaty of Waitangi. It was a brave action for a non-Māori leader to stand and deliver what he considered to be the right thing to do. Princess Mary Hospital was demolished and replaced with the new Connelly Unit as an Acute Mental Health ward.

'Dr Newman and the board took a risk in supporting this move because they saw that their failings to Māori far outweighed the backlash and the risk,' Amohaere comments. Despite strong vocal opposition, he pursued this avenue with Amohaere. The board's endorsement to allocate space on the top floor of the children's hospital for Amohaere and the Kāhui Kaumātua's vision was a milestone decision for the hospital and future Māori health initiatives.

It was to be the world's very first family support unit within a hospital system.[23]

*

In late 1989, Amohaere was appointed Tumuaki Atawhai – Manager Māori Health, a newly created bicultural manager position. The Kāhui Kaumātua were recognised as volunteering elders. When Bill Tāpuke raised the question with the Kāhui Kaumātua about a name for this new unit, Canon John Tamahori coined the phrase 'Te Whānau Atawhai' (the family of caring people). This was to become the formal title of the hospital's Māori Health Service. At the time the name was conferred, Canon Tamahori predicted that this entity would in time speak for itself. 'While Māori families' experiences in the hospitals of the past were not warm and friendly,' he exclaimed, 'so Te Whānau Atawhai will represent everything they want hospitals to be.' This was a profound statement and one that has always stayed with Amohaere.

Te Whānau Atawhai ki Princess Mary was officially launched in October of 1990 at a special gathering of more than a hundred people. It would become a central entity encompassing the Kāhui Kaumātua, Amohaere as Tumuaki and volunteers, with the ability to employ others in the future. The years Amohaere had worked as the cultural parent liaison officer, initially regarded as a support position with no real teeth and in a sometimes obstructive environment, had paid off. Amohaere and the kaumātua now felt there was a sense of full acceptance of Māori participation at a decision-making level in the hospital.

Architects began to draw up plans to make space for Te Whānau Atawhai on the seventh floor. Because this was a ground-breaking initiative, there were no set guidelines or procedures to run by. For Amohaere it was an exercise in innovation. 'The architects asked many questions about the cultural expectations for the spaces to include in the building process. We had to be creative.'

She was able to contribute to the look of the children's rooms, the colour schemes, the furnishings and space to include the needs of families. Amohaere recalls debates in those meetings as to whether to build the new hospital out at Middlemore or at the current Auckland Hospital site. The Whānau Room, an accommodation centre on the top floor of the building, was included in the plans and so too was the additional 'home away from home' facility to become known as Ronald McDonald House. This would offer families facing a challenging time additional accommodation and a private space. Amohaere was appointed a member of the steering committee for Ronald McDonald House, which was opened in 1994.

During earlier Kāhui Kaumātua meetings about the building of the new children's hospital, a number of important subjects arose. One was the notion of inviting mana whenua (the local tribal authority) to turn the soil before any building commenced on the hospital grounds. This also meant ascertaining who would officiate at the blessing for the opening ceremony of the finished hospital. These were ideas foreign to the thinking of the Pākehā executives and planners. When asked why mana whenua should be present at the soil turning ceremony, Amohaere explained to the board and architects how the whenua itself had a history that reached far beyond the time that the hospital was built on it. For that reason, the guardians of the local tribal territory deserved to be offered the right to bless the land in their own way for this new purpose.

As a result, Ngāti Whātua was recognised as the mana whenua and given the right to put the head of the spade into the ground first. This ceremony at the building site took place on 8 May 1988, the year the government finally decided to fund the hospital's construction after it had been proposed seven years earlier.[24]

All the Auckland tribes plus urban tribal representatives from out of the district were invited to participate on that important occasion. Because the hospital administered medical care to people from all tribes and nationalities, it was also considered fitting that all the tribes in the country should be represented. The dawn ceremony was held in the pouring rain. Canon John Tamahori officiated and translated for attending staff, many of whom were emotionally touched by the proceedings. For many, it was the first time they had attended any type of public ceremony driven by tikanga Māori.

In November 1989, the Kāhui Kaumātua were invited to attend the 'topping-off' ceremony. This was a modern variant of an ancient European builders' religious rite held when the last roof beam of a building structure is put in place to appease the tree spirits displaced in its construction.

The impressive 185-bed building was designed to be space efficient and to appeal specifically to children. It was characterised by pastel colours, woollen carpets throughout the wards and waiting rooms and space for children's artworks on the walls. At $79 million, it was the most expensive and complex building in New Zealand at the time.[25] It was also the first New Zealand hospital built exclusively for children and young people.

The new hospital was opened on 18 November 1991 at a large dawn dedication ceremony administered by Canon John Tamahori and the Kāhui Kaumātua. Canon Tamahori had organised fourteen ministers to dedicate the building – two placed on each of the seven floors. As they walked through the wards, they all recited karakia simultaneously to complete the blessing of the building. Amohaere remembers it as a truly magnificent day for Māori and Pākehā partnership in this organisation.

'It was a sight to behold, witnessing fourteen ministers chanting prayers through the building at the same time. The sound wafted down the centre of the hospital, to the amazement of the largely Pākehā medical fraternity gathered.'

*

Amohaere worked alongside Sir Bob Harvey (who in 1992 became Mayor of Waitakere and a member of the Starship Foundation), the then public relations officer for the project. One of the important tasks for this project was to consult with different groups on a possible name for the hospital. Finding themselves in a lift with a young child one day, they asked him what he thought of the new hospital. The youngster replied, 'It's like a huge starship!' Bob and Amohaere looked at each other. It was a 'Eureka!' moment and they put 'Starship' on the board table for debate as a potential hospital name. There was caution at board level. Some felt the name could imply the idea of a deceased child being sent to heaven on a starship. However, after some deliberation the board decided to run with it, and Starship Children's Hospital was formally given its name in 1992.

The seventh floor space allocated for Te Whānau Atawhai ki Auckland Hospital was situated between the oncology department and general management. The area consisted of office space, a common room, kitchen, three bedroom facilities and a laying-out room for the dead. These resources were managed through protocols set by the Kāhui Kaumātua. The unit's mission statement was to 'Provide Māori Health Services to improve the quality of life for Māori and all other people in Tāmaki Makau Rau'. The kaupapa of Te Whānau Atawhai was 'whanaungatanga – awhi, manaaki, atawhai'[26] (create a sense of family – embrace, support, care). The core principles of Te Whānau Atawhai developed by the elders were to implement and develop a whānau concept within the healing process for children and their families; develop cultural awareness and strengthen relationships with medical/nursing staff and other disciplines; provide a link to the community for ongoing support; and enable the kaupapa to permeate the existing service.[27]

Later, Te Whānau Atawhai Māori Health Services Unit, as a member of the senior management team within Auckland hospitals, contributed to continuous quality improvements in the delivery of health services to Māori consumers. It also helped to encourage the greater participation of Māori at all levels of health service delivery and to address training and development needs of Māori employees.

Te Whānau Atawhai sought to express its partnership role through the notion of whanaungatanga, building strong relationships between staff, patients and whānau and acknowledging their whakapapa (genealogy), whānau (family, extended family), hapū (wider extended family) and iwi (tribe) connections. These principles aimed to remove barriers to appropriate care, rehabilitation and wellbeing.

In Amohaere's experience, nurses did not have good communication skills. Many were young and ignorant of Māori and Pacific languages and were even known to yell at patients if there was a communication breakdown. She felt they came across as being very stern and almost always considered themselves correct. In turn, Māori people were intimidated by the environment and never spoke their mind truthfully. There were no formal greetings that Māori were so accustomed to in common life and no reo or tikanga-based engagement in the hospitals. These offended Māori patients and families and created unresponsiveness. It was something Te Whānau Atawhi attempted to rectify.

However, full acceptance of Te Whānau Atawhai's right to exist was still under fire, despite the unit already being in place on the top floor. A turning point came in 1991 when Amohaere was invited to address the Medical Grand Round. This was a regular forum where guest presenters lectured on issues with implications for practising physicians and specialists. It was an opportunity to discuss and debate specific medical cases with all in-house staff and peers. It was also regarded as a fearsome round table of critique and scrutiny. The audience didn't pull any punches. This meeting was to be held in the conference room on the top floor where Te Whānau Atawhai had been established. It was an opportunity for Amohaere to inform the hospital medical professionals what her role as Tumuaki Atawhai entailed and why it was imperative that it continue.

'There were around eighty doctors in the gathering, some supported our move and others were still opposed. Many had never engaged with Māori at this level. I was introduced by Dr Newman and asked to share about Te Whānau Atawhai. Sheepishly, I began with a mihi, then continued to explain my experiences stepping onto the floor in the wards.'

There was a high level of curiosity amongst the doctors, and for Amohaere, standing before them all was daunting to say the least. 'I was told nearly 60 percent of the patients in the wards were my people, so it was appropriate to have a Māori speak to the senior members. One hour seemed like an eternity,' she remembers.

On that day, Dr Stewart Fergusson, a strong adversary and an intimidating force, sat right in the front row. Amohaere was therefore greatly surprised when, at the conclusion of her presentation, he stood up and encouraged the entire gathering to give her a standing ovation. He had never heard the Māori world explored in this manner. 'You took it to the heart of the people's needs,' he said. There were no further questions from the floor, and at that point, Amohaere knew there was full buy-in from the doctors.

From that day, doctors from all specialist areas asked that Amohaere attend their meetings or walk through their wards to point out discrepancies from her cultural point of view. Amohaere always responded to these requests. As far as she was concerned, a face seen is a voice heard. It was all-important to build trust amongst the ranks of decision makers. In her own way, she knew she was accountable to them all as well as to the patients. 'We got so chummy we'd touch each other when we'd meet and often kiss hello in the wards – something that would never have happened previously in such a sterile environment.'

This expression of aroha changed attitudes and slowly infiltrated many areas of the hospital, not only between staff, but also in the wards where a more homely atmosphere was created. Amohaere formed close relationships with her peers, as a kind of mother or a sister figure, placing a korowai of aroha around people. But caring for the child patients was paramount.

'Creating a state of wellness, in my mind, included a safe environment for the children by creating a homely feeling to enhance and elevate their wellness, and ultimately hoping that they would go home earlier.'

NINE

Expanding Horizons

One group Amohaere greatly admired for their loving work with the children in Princess Mary Hospital and later at Starship were the grandparent volunteers. This was a core of ten to fifteen women who substituted as caring grandparents for those children in the wards who had no visitors.

'They would visit the children daily, bathe them, read them stories and take them for pushchair rides through the corridors. All were Pākehā except for one shy old Māori kuia, Aunty Mate. She would search me out when she was on site, carrying the Māori babies in her arms.' Amohaere applauded their work and saw great value in making strong relationships with these kinds of groups.

Te Whānau Atawhai functioned in a similar way, for the same cause, but from a Māori cultural perspective. In its daily running, Te Whānau Atawhai's Whānau Room was frequented by Māori elders as volunteers – kuia and kaumātua rostered to be on hand for the children and the visiting families. The order of the day always began with karakia at 8.30 a.m. followed by mihi, waiata and a briefing. These caring pākeke (elders) were essential to creating an environment of wellness, so much so that when children had to go home, many would cry to stay with them.

Volunteer kaumātua Brownie Williams saw the Whānau Atawhai unit as a 'mini-mobile-marae stalking the wards of Auckland's hospitals, trying to ensure that the medical system is sensitive to the needs of its Māori consumers'.[1] His role was as simple as 'sitting at the shoulder of a patient's relatives, giving them the courage to ask the questions they needed answered. It may mean calling Māori outpatients who have missed a clinic appointment because they can't afford the transport and are too ashamed to admit it, then picking them up in a board car, [and] promising clinical staff, they're going to be late, but they'll be here.'²

In addition to the pākeke volunteers, broadening the services of Te Whānau Atawhai meant finding more competent Māori workers. Amohaere had been contacted by Mavis Tuoro and Toby Curtis from the Auckland Institute of Technology, who ran a kaupapa Māori social services certificate programme. They were searching for placement opportunities for their Māori students. Mavis had previously been unable to place students in the hospital social work department because there was no belief that her programme had the right accreditation to warrant providing placements. Amohaere sought the support of her ally Mary Futter, and it was Nurse Futter who was responsible for opening the door to kaupapa Māori placements with the first student beginning in August 1990.³ From that time on, there were twice-yearly student placements. At the end of their allotted time, some of the students continued to volunteer in the unit. In time, when positions became available within Te Whānau Atawhai, they filled some of them.

Te Whānau Atawhai Annual Report for 1992 noted that staff in the unit consisted of four full-time kaiatawhai who worked closely with a team of kaumātua, kuia kaitiaki and volunteer kaiatawhai.⁴ The Kaiatawhai team had progressed to working in Auckland Hospital, Starship and the Acute Mental Health ward, on a sixteen-hour roster with a twenty-four-hour on-call service, maintaining the 'whanaungatanga' kaupapa in its broadest meaning.⁵

According to Te Whānau Atawhai management plan for 1990–1991, the full team of kaiatawhai comprised the following people:

Kaumātua
Canon John Tamahori (Ngāti Porou)
Danny Tumahai (Ngāti Whātua)
Jack Wihongi (Tai Tokerau, Ngā Puhi, Tainui)
Ruby Gray (Ngāti Whātua)

Chairperson
Brownie Williams (Ngāti Awa)

Members
Bill Tāpuke (Taranaki)
Dean Rua (Ngāti Whātua)

Whaea
Mahia Wallace (Tūhourangi)
Monica Rogers (Tainui)

Kuia
Amelia Oppenheimer (Tai Tokerau)
Wiki Henskes (Tainui)

Tumuaki Atawhai
Amohaere Gardiner Tangitu (Te Arawa, Ngāti Awa)

Advisory Group
Phyllis Tangitu (Te Arawa)
Sam Rolleston (Ngāti Ranginui, Ngāti Rangi)

Volunteers
Harata Tahere (Tai Tokerau)
Ngāpine Brown (Te Aupouri)
Hana Taylor (Ngāti Wai)

Kaitiaki
Brownie Williams (Ngāti Awa)
Aronia Ahomiro (Te Arawa)
Graeme Smith (Tainui)
Harata Apii (Ngā Puhi)

Salaried Kaiatawhai Workers
Jocelyn Jacobs (Ngāti Ranginui)
Vyna Wiki (Te Arawa)
Adelaide Waata (Te Arawa)
Lullita Samuels (Tainui)
Richard Rātapu (Ngāti Porou)

Kaiatawhai had a positive working relationship with doctors and nursing staff, providing cultural advice to them. They also sought accommodation for families from out of the Auckland area, and where needed, they ensured the spiritual needs of patients and their families were provided for by making contact with ministers of their chosen religions.[6]

Follow-up with patients in the community was important. Linking up with Māori health community workers ensured the holistic needs of patients and their families were met. Kaiatawhai were involved in multidisciplinary meetings in Starship and also in several of the Auckland Hospital wards. This was regarded as a major achievement for Te Whānau Atawhai, which was often called to react to a situation rather than participating at the beginning of a process where any cultural transgressions could easily be foreseen and averted.[7]

In 1992, Ngāti Whātua ki Orākei requested that Te Whānau Atawhai extend its service into the Acute Mental Health Unit owing to the large number of Māori admissions there. Te Whānau Atawhai obliged, but it was a stretch. With charge nurses continually seeking the services of kaiatawhai at multidisciplinary meetings in Auckland Hospital, Starship and Mental Health Services, it was difficult for the small Te Whānau Atawhai team to participate fully. Its effectiveness came down to the committed combination of employed kaiatawhai and the volunteer services of the elders.[8] The projected goal for 1991–1992 was to increase the number of paid kaiatawhai positions.[9]

By 1992, Amohaere and her team had made inroads into areas such as the surgical theatres where the disposal of patients' limbs was deemed to be a concern.[10] Over time, liaison with Auckland Hospital Theatre Charge Nurse Sue Frost brought about change on this issue. Of particular importance, a protocol was established in 1992 for the return of limbs and tissue to the family for burial.[11] The undertaker was commissioned to create special containers for limbs, but a similar process was yet to be established for tissue.[12]

Amohaere was always concerned about the way the hospital treated families in mourning. When the wishes of whānau to grieve openly and prepare the tūpāpaku for burial were denied them by culturally insensitive hospital policies, she intuitively felt their pain. However, through education and promotion of cultural sensitivities, procedures for the care of tūpāpaku, the retrieval of body tissue by whānau and the blessing of bed spaces were introduced. Disposable body sheets for tūpāpaku was another initiative that grew out of the work of Te Whānau Atawhai.

Kaiatawhai were often called to support whānau pani (families in mourning). They were assisted in coming to terms with the coroner's processes and with their interaction with funeral directors.[13] Space was also set aside on Te Whānau Atawhai site for tūpāpaku to lie in state, when needed, before being taken by the whānau pani. Here all the necessary Māori ceremonies around death, common to iwi, could be carried out safely. This space was available to both Māori and non-Māori families.

For Amohaere and her staff, attending community and tribal hui was imperative. This was primarily to keep community ties alive, to network and to promote the bicultural services available within the hospital. They attended medical forums, Te Puni Kōkiri gatherings and tribal hui, not only in the Auckland region, but further afield in Rotorua, Whakatāne and Wellington. Listening to the voices of communities and iwi as to how they saw the administration of health care was vital for Te Whānau Atawhai's ability to be effective for its own people.

A growing awareness of bicultural expansion within all aspects of hospital life saw a number of new appointments made. To cover the increasing workload in the two hospitals, Amohaere and the team pushed for another bicultural officer who would be responsible to the Auckland Hospital General Manager. It would be a position similar to Amohaere's, but under her management. Anaru Kiira, the Māori Liaison Officer for Te Roopu Kai Ārahi Ki Te Ora, was later appointed as the Māori Health Manager at Auckland Hospital, with a daunting job description. Among other things, he was tasked to 'ensure quality health care outcomes through the interpretation and implementation of the Tiriti o Waitangi to positively reflect equity and tino rangatiratanga, and to promote understanding and communication with te iwi Māori'.[14]

Wally Te Ua became the first Māori chaplain for Starship Hospital – a first for any hospital in New Zealand. The Māori Anglican world was introduced into the hospital realm with clergy such as Hone Kaa, Muru Walters and Kito Pikaahu all playing a role in the wards over the years. This was considered a real coup at the time.

With the increase in demand for services came greater responsibilities and the need for more administration. Other new positions were created and filled. One was the Kaiwhiriwhiri (Administrator for Human Resources), a role designed by Amohaere, Karena Way and Airini Tukerangi to ensure that appointment procedures on the Auckland Hospital site were culturally appropriate.[15] The Kaiwhiriwhiri would be a bicultural representative on interview panels for new employees. This position would be essential also in the writing of new job descriptions and in the decision-making process.[16] The other administrative position was that of Kai Whakahaere – Kaiatawhai Supervisor.[17]

From 1991, Amohaere and Wi Keelan sat on the then newly formed New Zealand Healthcare Standards Surveying Committee, chaired by Pauline Kingi. This committee was formed to measure an organisation's cultural competencies within the health sector. Together, they created the standards and the levels of competency needed in the areas of culturally safe care, tikanga Māori, responsiveness, service and education training. Māori cultural competence was explained as specific requirements for best practice to assist advocates to provide services appropriate and acceptable to Māori. These competencies required a commitment to continuous improvement through ongoing planning, education, training and review. Dr Mason Durie notes that cultural competence had to do with the 'acquisition of skills to achieve a better understanding of other cultures'. The goal of culturally competent care was to 'improve relationships and thereby achieve better clinical results'.[18]

In early 1992, when moves were taken to reconfigure and separate the Area Health Boards into Regional Health Agencies and Crown Health Enterprises,

Amohaere as Tumuaki Atawhai and Te Whānau Atawhai had to reaffirm their effectiveness under this restructure. The Crown Health Enterprise structure was committed to biculturalism, and this was reiterated in the new Auckland Hospital Statement of Function.[19] Te Whānau Atawhai chair Brownie Williams sought assurances under the new structure that its management and support functions would continue to service the needs of the Māori people and foster and implement biculturalism.[20] Te Whānau Atawhai and its tumuaki position were eventually rolled over into the Crown Health Enterprise structure.

*

Through all this change and reorganisation, the needs of patients were still paramount. That never changed. The unit still had two sixteen-hour rostered shifts operating on both the Starship and the main Auckland hospital sites. After midnight, one of the team was always on call till 7 a.m. In September 1992, there was still only a limited staff of six to cover the growing services.[21]

Orientation training and education on the Treaty of Waitangi, biculturalism and competencies in culturally appropriate care became a major focus for Amohaere and tangata tiriti (people of the Treaty) colleague Karena Way. They organised and delivered education sessions with the support of the Training and Development Service of Human Resources, Auckland Hospital.[22] Due to the rapid staff turnover within the Auckland hospitals and teaching and research responsibilities, orientation and training on these core values needed to be continuously taught, updated and reviewed. Early in the piece, the

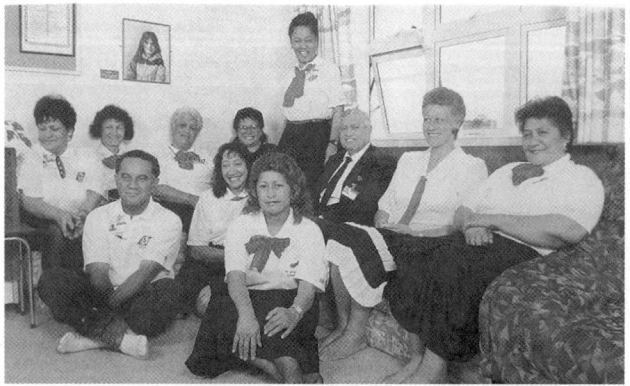

Te Whānau Atawhai staff, pictured here in their new facility on the seventh level of Starship Hospital.
SOURCED FROM *TE WHĀNAU ATAWHAI, A NEW INITIATIVE IN HEALTH PROVISION*, 1993

Kāhui Kaumātua set cultural care protocols and competencies in place and sought to put these into staff performance assessments associated with cultural interactions.

The orientation seminars to present the bicultural policy were rolled out for all the nurses and support staff and were included in the medical and mental health programmes. The seminars also introduced the roles of the tumuaki atawhai, the kaiatawhai and the kaiwhiriwhiri and the practice of cultural safety to all on site. Monthly Treaty of Waitangi workshops provided perspectives on history, culture and the Treaty for non-Māori and explained the rationale for cultural safety. Te Whānau Atawhai introduced their kaupapa and practice and explained how they and staff could work together to provide the highest quality customer service.

Amohaere, Karena Way and available kaiatawhai also delivered regular mini seminars on kawa whakaruruhau (cultural safety) to in-service sessions organised by the clinical nurse specialists in the wards. These kawa whakaruruhau sessions were extended outside the wards to health staff and students in the polytechnics and medical schools. Additional individual education or advice sessions were provided in response to ongoing requests from nurses, social workers and medical and management staff. For Te Whānau Atawhai hands-on workers, training was delivered by Amohaere, elders and the new supervisor with input from the Starship Clinical Nurse Specialist and Auckland Hospital Training and Development.[23] Māori language classes for non-speaking staff were run by Mita Makiha.[24]

In 1993, the activities of Te Whānau Atawhai fell into two arenas. The functional roles focused directly on strategic planning and development, while the service arm of the unit revolved around core services to the child patients and their whānau. The service arena included kaiatawhai – salaried workers involved in direct client servicing; kaitiaki – volunteer workers as assistants to the kaiatawhai; community liaison – establishing community links and facilitating direct service involvement; whare hāpai – focusing on Māori health and biculturalism training and development; and whare mate – facilities where the proper cultural bereavement customs could be carried out.[25]

A paper written by Amohaere, Brian Henderson and Karena Way and delivered to an Australasian Paediatrics Conference in Wellington in 1993 outlined a bicultural approach to paediatric care using the example of Te Whānau Atawhai. By this time, there were three full-time salaried workers and five unpaid volunteers in the unit. In the newly formed Paediatrics Intensive Care Unit (PICU), Te Whānau Atawhai provided emotional and physical support during emergency calls to patients and families, supported families of dying children, provided physical comforts such as an overnight bed and tea/coffee facilities for parents, assisted in liaising with community networks and social facilities, educated PICU staff in areas of cultural difference and helped explain to relatives the necessity for some of the PICU procedures and protocols. The paper stressed that Te Whānau Atawhai, as a support group, were not in opposition to the Social Services Department but that the two units worked together to provide benefits to families of sick children.[26]

At the conference, Amohaere was accompanied by kaumātua hospital volunteers. Her presentation began with lights dimmed, the sound of a kōauau (traditional flute) and the recital of a tauparapara (chant) to create a mood and context for what was to follow. Her efforts won the award for the best presentation at the conference, highlighting, as they did, the notion of a bicultural view on health care as a priority for the future.

*

All through this period, whānau, hapū, iwi and other medical institutions began to seek out Amohaere about the bicultural processes she and Te Whānau Atawhai had implemented at the Auckland Hospital site.

The Auckland Area Health Board extended its boundary to include Greenlane Hospital, and this, in turn, extended Amohaere's role. The quality assurance nurse for Greenlane invited her to visit the paediatric department, in particular the cardiac and respiratory units that many Māori children were referred to. Amohaere visited the wards to look in on Māori patients and their families and identify their needs. Patient advocates had already been set in place, but delivery of culturally appropriate care for Māori was still to be reviewed. Greenlane was a specialist hospital but, like Princess Mary Hospital, needed to upskill staff in the knowledge and understanding of cultural safety and practice.

The impetus for this request may have emerged out of the findings of the Cartwright Inquiry report of 1988. Creating a relationship with Amohaere and the Whānau Atawhai unit was extremely advantageous to fulfilling some of the recommendations of this report for Greenlane.

The Cartwright Inquiry was a judicial review into unethical research conducted at Auckland University's postgraduate school of Obstetrics and Gynaecology at National Women's Hospital, Greenlane. Phillida Bunkle and Sandra Coney's article 'An Unfortunate Experiment' published in *Metro* magazine in 1987 highlighted how 'women with precancerous carcinoma in situ of the cervix (CIS), and some with micro-invasive cancer of the cervix or vaginal vault had, without their knowledge, received repeated diagnostic biopsies and cervical smears, but had been left untreated or undertreated in order to study the extent to which these lesions developed into invasive cancer. The result was that many developed invasive cancer and some died'.[27] The government of the day responded by setting up a judicial inquiry headed by District Court Judge Silvia Cartwright.

The findings and recommendations sparked off a massive controversy. The report found the allegations to be correct. It was critical of the 'objectification of patients' that implied 'inhuman treatment'.[28]

While Judge Cartwright's report was specific to National Women's Hospital, it highlighted a number of areas strongly applicable to Amohaere's personal experience with hospitals and to her own position at that time as Princess Mary Hospital's Manager Māori Health. The judge spoke to specific aspects of improvement, covering patients' rights, patient advocates, formal and informal consents, access to Māori and other cultural interpreters and translators, communication, privacy and dignity.[29]

In response to this, Amohaere's relationship with managers and staff at Greenlane soon saw the establishment of a series of staff seminars on the subject of 'difference'. Senior nurses desired a greater level of competent cultural practice. They knew staff needed to know what it looked like in action, so a series of cultural awareness seminars was incorporated into the training for the Greenlane and National Women's hospital staff. To Amohaere, the need to set up structures for the provision of culturally safe care in both these institutions had been evident for many years, especially as Māori hospital admission rates for circulatory diseases and complications of pregnancy and birth were significantly higher than those for non-Māori.[30]

Funding would be needed to expand the service to fully integrate Te Whānau Atawhai within Greenlane and National Women's Hospitals. In 1994, Amohaere identified what initial preparations would be needed for integration. It was a huge task, involving a needs analysis to prioritise areas where placement of kaiatawhai would be most effective within the management and medical personnel of both hospitals. From modest beginnings, Amohaere's role had expanded enormously as the seeds of cultural awareness and safe practice began to take root within the wider hospital system.

Families deeply appreciated Te Whānau Atawhai's services. 'We were taken care of from the moment we arrived. We came on a weekend. The Te Whānau Atawhai people showed us the hospital, explained the system and encouraged us,' one family shared. Another parent said, 'We felt simply better for being greeted by the words "kia ora"' and yet another commented that 'It's almost like being at home.'[31] Of particular importance to these whānau was the knowledge that there would be follow-up visits by Te Whānau Atawhai through their support networks.

This was considered a radical type of service for its time and attracted attention from many medical organisations and other interested parties, including visiting celebrities. National and international guest visits to Starship were common. The regard health officials had for Te Whānau Atawhai was shown when a request for Charles, Prince of Wales, to visit the unit was accepted by the committee in 1994. Toby Curtis and Amohaere organised a formal pōwhiri for the Prince to be performed by the kaiatawhai team, despite the many constraints and formalities of a royal visit. Prince Charles was then escorted by Amohaere through Te Whānau Atawhai and the children's wards to meet the children and their families. Prince Charles showed a genuine interest in the philosophy of the unit and its operations. In speaking of Prince Charles's visit, Toby Curtis, then chairman of Te Whānau Atawhai, wrote to the Chief Executive of Auckland Healthcare that, 'the position occupied by Te Whānau Atawhai throughout the proceedings was a clear illustration of the practice of biculturalism within this institution'.[32] A similar visit by famous Pakistani cricketer Imran Khan also put Te Whānau Atawhai in the limelight. Canon Tamahori stressed the importance of good public relations, such as these visits, to further the kaupapa of Te Whānau Atawhai as a working model for other hospitals. Amohaere remembers how he often reiterated the adage: 'Mā ngā mahi e mōhiotia ai' ('By the work we will be known').[33]

*

An increasing workload for Amohaere and Te Whānau Atawhai plus the constant and sometimes ridiculous changes in the political reorganisation of the health system forced the creation of new strategies to fit in with new governance structures. The Auckland Area Health Board was transformed into a Crown Health Enterprise (CHE) and was to be re-configured into the Auckland District Health Board, funded by the Regional Health Authority (RHA). This meant the board would geographically encompass the services at Starship, Auckland Hospital and include Greenlane Hospital and National Women's. Whatever this new entity would look like, it would need a governance relationship with Māori and a new Māori strategic plan.

The Minister of Health's August 1992 statement introducing the new RHA's purchasing plan required providers to have a community focus, a culturally sensitive perspective, accountability to consumers, an innovative and flexible approach to support services, and the skills to responsibly use the financial resources.[34] In response to the changes, a new Māori health strategy was set to be developed from 1993 to satisfy RHA requirements and to further maintain tikanga 'best practice' within the future restructure. Amohaere as Manager Māori Health Management for Te Whānau Atawhai and Naida Pou (Glavish) as Manager Māori Health Management Te Takiwā Toka Oranga combined to develop a Māori health management plan to assist Auckland Healthcare Services Ltd, the entity in charge of all Auckland regional hospitals, 'to achieve sustainable health services to Aucklanders and especially Māori as tangata whenua'.[35]

This proposed strategic plan was entitled *He Kamaka Oranga Strategic Plan 1993/1994, Māori Health Management Developments to the Year 2000*.[36] It proposed that Te Whānau Atawhai would manage Child Health, Auckland Hospital, Greenlane Hospital, Women's Health (National Women's Hospital) and the Connelly Unit (Acute Mental Health). Te Takiwā Toka Oranga would manage Community Health Services (Health Promotion Education, Sexual Health, National Audio, and Ngā Purapura), Mental Health Services (Manaaki House, Maranga Health, Manawanui), Head Injuries (Sutherland Unit), and Waiheke and Aotea Islands health care. Focus of the plan on Māori management and leadership would be advanced from within the chief executive's office and other key hospital service areas.[37]

The mission statement of *He Kamaka Oranga* was to 'Provide sustainable Māori health management to improve the quality of life for Māori and all other people in Tāmaki Makau Rau while preserving those visions and qualities unique to Māori', with its key values still being 'Whanaungatanga – Āwhina, Manaaki, Atawhai'.[38] The structure of Māori health management would be directly accountable to the Auckland Healthcare chief executive with support drawn from Te Whānau Atawhai and Te Rūnanga o Ngāti Whātua kaumātua and kuia. It would also seek to create strategic alliances with Te Puni Kōkiri, Manatū Hauora, Te Rūnanga o Ngāti Whātua, Taura Here, Te Whānau o Waipareira, Huakina Development Trust, Rangapū Hauora Tumatanui, and Mana Hauora a Rohe o Te Raki – all organisations within the new geographic greater Auckland region.[39]

To succeed, there needed to be an agreed partnership protocol between Māori Health Management and Auckland Healthcare, a review of existing resources to increase Māori managers' capability to deliver health care, the introduction of a measureable training plan and a belief in the kaupapa.[40]

'It was stated,' Amohaere remembers, 'that this was the first major "mainstream enhancement strategy" of its kind nationally.'

After presenting the strategy to staff and community health workers on the Tāmaki Marae at Ihumātao, Amohaere, Toby Curtis and Naida went on to present *He Kamaka Oranga* to the management and staff of North Health (the Northern Regional Health Authority) in March, 1994.[41] *He Kamaka Oranga* would soon take on a life of its own within the system. Auckland hospitals were growing in their acceptance of Treaty obligations, biculturalism, cultural safety and the place of Māori services, particularly in the area of nursing policy and standards of practice.[42]

The mechanics for the meaningful implementation of cultural safety with a clear acceptance of spiritual, physical and cultural dimensions of care were now firmly fixed within the system.[43] The terms of reference in the nurses' policy made clear guidelines around the rights of patients and whānau to culturally sensitive care, shared decision making between whānau and the health provider, ongoing staff training in cultural safety practice, acceptance of te reo Māori and other languages in all communications, inclusion of the tumuaki atawhai in health care plans across the board and involvement of Te Whānau Atawhai as professional assistants in admissions, care, discharge and deaths.[44] Specific practices around non-verbal behaviours, blessing rooms, respecting patients' bodies, retention of limbs, linen, food and consents were listed as issues of cultural sensitivity.

*

During 1994, Amohaere sensed a change in the air, not only in the mechanics of the health system, but also in her own personal life journey. It had always been her dream to someday return to her own people in Whakatāne to work, but also to regain something lost. 'I wanted to return home while my mother was still alive and seek something of my own identity that I had lost since living my entire married life in Auckland. The call home was almost unrelenting.' The only question was 'When should I move?'

She could see the writing on the wall. There was a major shift brewing in the politics of future governance and leadership within the Māori health sector in Tāmaki Makaurau. The prominent rise of Ngāti Whātua as mana whenua in the region would see their relationship with local institutions, including the Auckland hospitals, soon take precedence over other internal Māori-run health organisations like Te Whānau Atawhai. As she and Te Whānau Atawhai Kāhui

Kaumātua saw it, 'this was probably part of the natural progression of the Treaty and bicultural training now becoming a reality'.

Amohaere spoke to the Kāhui Kaumātua about her wish to make moves homeward, and they were supportive of her desire. She then raised this subject with Ngāti Whātua elders Doc Wikiriwhi, Danny Tumahai, the kuia Ruby Gray and Ann Pihama. She had served with them all on the Kāhui Kaumātua council. Amohaere suggested they should probably look to filling her shoes with someone from Ngāti Whātua. 'Doc was grateful for the inclusion of Ngāti Whātua as mana whenua in the health services sector over the years and was happy for whatever decision I would make,' she remembers.

On 20 August 1994, Amohaere left Auckland Hospital with the sanction of the Kāhui Kaumātua and made a crucial move to the Bay of Plenty.

Amohaere has been credited with making Auckland hospitals more user-friendly for Māori and initiating an advocacy service for Māori patients, Māori staff recruitment policies and cultural safety training for doctors and nurses. Looking back, she realises how difficult it all was, especially having limited education and continually coming up against brick walls. She just saw the need for a whānau support unit. It was a priority for families who had nowhere to stay, wash or eat while they were visiting their children. 'Recovery of the child depends on whānau involvement and I wanted to ensure the needs of the whānau were taken care of so they could focus on their sick tamariki.'[45]

In the space of seven years from Amohaere's entry into the hospital world, a great deal of political and practical change had occurred at so many levels. Amohaere and her supporters had slowly broken new ground especially with the establishment of Te Whānau Atawhai in 1990.

After Amohaere's departure, Te Whānau Atawhai was integrated into He Kamaka Oranga (HKO) Māori Health, which became the over-arching strategy for the Auckland District Health Board (ADHB). The essential aim of HKO was improving the health and wellbeing of this area's Māori population.[46] Along with this change and amidst a tribal power struggle, the multi-tribal entity of the Te Whānau Atawhai Kāhui Kaumātua was eventually dissolved – to the dismay of many.

It was the end of one season for the hospital but the beginning of a new destiny for Amohaere.

TEN

Hunga Manaaki

Looking for an opportunity to move closer to home, in 1994 Amohaere applied for a position at Rotorua Hospital. Lakeland Health was looking for an iwi consultant to begin creating a working relationship between Te Arawa and Tūwharetoa tribes and to produce a Māori health strategy for the hospitals in the Central Plateau region. She was offered the job. The shift towards her own tribal roots was now becoming more of a reality.

Not only was Amohaere moving to a new job closer to whānau, she was also making a bold move towards reclaiming her own personal identity. She changed her name by deed poll from Judith Amohaere Ngaropo back to her maiden surname, Tangitu. This name change along with the deeper reclamation of her own Māoritanga was not well received by her husband who strongly voiced his opinions with statements like 'You belong at home looking after the kids,' and 'That Māori world is worth nothing. It will never get you anywhere.' However, her children were now living their own lives, and she felt free to make decisions for her own life. She eventually separated from her husband, Sam, but never divorced him.

Amohaere's mother cautioned her against the move, saying, 'Your own people will be the most critical of you. Do you really want to come home?' On top of that, she counselled her daughter that if she was looking to bring back old customary ideas, she must put boundaries in place to hold the customs properly. None of her mother's warnings lessened Amohaere's strong resolve to return home, but she knew that by taking up the Rotorua job offer, she would have to tread carefully, with humility and under a mantle of kaumatuatanga.

The iwi consultant was to undertake a full cultural audit of the organisation.[1] This included consulting with the Ngāti Tūwharetoa tribal group and Te Arawa confederacy of tribes. Tūwharetoa had just recently come out from under the Waikato District Health Board and were now reconstituted under the Lakes District Health Board. Additionally, in 1993, Lakeland Health had publicly stated it was committed to establishing long-term relationships with iwi who recognised the value of this kind of relationship and the impact it might have on Māori health status. A connection would be developed between Lakeland Health and Te Mana Hauora o Te Arawa, the officially mandated Māori health authority in Te Arawa tribal region.[2]

Lakes District Health Board records two major factors that contributed to this desire for these relationships. Firstly, 40 percent of those accessing hospital or community services were Māori. Secondly, the concerns of iwi about the delivery of health care services to Māori had to be considered.[3] This included the notion of culturally appropriate health services, something DHB chair Stewart Edward had always believed in.[4] While Lakeland Health and local Māori organisations knew 'what' they had to move forward with, they needed someone to spearhead the 'how'.

Amohaere was apprehensive about taking on the role, knowing full well she was an unknown face in the region. She would have to pull together local elders to carry herself and the kaupapa before the people of Tūwharetoa. It was a daunting task to say the least. She knew she would have to stand on the mana of her grandmother Amohaere, an original member of the Women's Health League in Rotorua, and work with integrity amongst the people to maintain her namesake's mana in the region. Her biggest question was, 'How am I going to consult with Tūwharetoa?'

Working with iwi in their own territories was a new dynamic for Amohaere who had only known an urban multi-tribal arena. This journey would be fraught with danger as each iwi was fiercely independent of others and possessed, on the whole, its own independent health services.

Amohaere's initial thought was to form a Kāhui Kaumātua. 'As far as I was concerned, the elders were the key to uniting the people.' An approach was made to Uncle Joe Malcolm, Tūtānekai Kinita and others, who called a gathering of the 'eight beating hearts of Rangitihi' – a term given to the tribal descendants of the eight sons of Rangitihi, a senior Te Arawa ancestor. Gunner Raharuhi, Kawana Nepia, Ani Paul, Sam Hahunga and others all came together to meet in the Rotorua Hospital boardroom. Amohaere introduced herself and explained the purpose of the gathering – to find an eldership that would accompany her to Tūwharetoa.

Ngāti Pikiao took up the cause of accompanying Amohaere to Tūrangi and Tokaanu and creating introductions with Tūwharetoa. Initially, however, there was suspicion, and Amohaere remembers it being hard work. Tūwharetoa and Te Arawa were totally independent tribes, despite being under the same district health region. It was to take time and a number of visits to establish some kind of relationship. As a result, Whakapūmautanga (Darkie) Downes, a well-respected and wise elder, agreed to become the Tūwharetoa representative on the District Health Board Kāhui Kaumātua.

This was the beginning of her consultation process, which then expanded to everyone from hauora providers, Te Puni Kōkiri and other iwi and hapū in the region. There was general hesitancy as the groups sought to understand the kaupapa of Amohaere's brief and what they could expect to receive out of these relationships. Eventually, a Kāhui Kaumātua eldership was created with iwi and hapū representatives on board.

Amohaere was to ascertain the health needs and aspirations of the iwi, with the details to be delivered to Lakes District Health Board in an iwi consultant's report. She was there to empower the tribes and whānau by reporting to Lakeland Health their needs and making suggestions as to how to meet their requirements.

As part of the consultancy, an extensive questionnaire surveying the clinical journey of Māori patients' experiences within the hospital, from entry to exit, was carried out. Patients were asked to evaluate everything from the food and the environment to the delivery of services by nurses, doctors and social workers. The survey lasted eight months and revealed the need for a lot more application of culturally sensitive care when dealing with patients. Of course, there was nothing new in this for Amohaere.

Delivered to the board in 1995, the report presented a greater picture of how the local services were perceived by Māori, and this information would be used to develop and implement a better approach to achieving Māori needs and aspirations. The report recommended a five-year strategic plan with suggestions for mechanisms to make hospital services at Rotorua more culturally appropriate. This included creating the position of a Manager Māori Health answerable to the Lakes District Health Board. Similar to Te Whānau Atawhai model, this position would sit alongside a Kāhui Kaumātua of Te Arawa and Tūwharetoa representatives. The Manager Māori Health would run a team of workers specific to this unit to implement the policies of good tikanga practice and service on the hospital floor.

The allocation of services was to be contracted out to Te Mana Hauora o Te Arawa, the mandated Māori health provider for the region, and funds would be allocated for the full function of this system. Amohaere felt that developing bicultural policies would also strengthen the interaction and relationship between Lakeland Health and the Māori population it served.

At the time, Māori services in the hospital were minimal. It was common, for example, to find Māori health coordinators stretched to capacity working across the entire hospital. Rotorua Hospital's first Māori Health Coordinator was former nurse Teresa Winiata, who worked in the role from the late 1980s until her retirement in the mid-1990s.

Amohaere's recommendations were incorporated into the District Health Plan, and Amohaere was asked at the behest of the Kāhui Kaumātua to take up the position of Manager, Māori Health in order to build the structures described in the summary of the report. The major difference between setting up this system in Rotorua and her years in Auckland was the fact that there were only two core tribes and one mana whenua group to associate with. Also, the education programmes required for this system to work were already in place. Another difference for Amohaere was that she was not required to walk the wards as she had in Auckland. While this model was based on Te Whānau Atawhai unit in Auckland, the added details of its management and boundaries were set by the local tribes themselves. 'It was an adaptation of a proven service,' Amohaere comments.

A new entity, Hunga Manaaki, the name coined by well-known Rotorua kuia Bubbles Mihinui, emerged. 'This kuia was strict, spoke her mind, but always had wise words,' Amohaere remembers. She always sought her advice concerning the Māori way of approaching wellness, something Bubbles always laughed about. 'The day you know what the Māori way is can you come and tell me, Amohaere?' she'd laugh. There is no 'one Māori way' but more a series of common tikanga adjustable to a local region, Amohaere believes. 'That's why any forward progress in health strategy couldn't be modelled solely on one particular way but had to be collectively agreed to and adapted to fit the local tribal boundaries.'

In its early stages Hunga Manaaki was to provide culturally appropriate care at the hospital funded under Lakeland Health, Rotorua Hospital. A key goal was simply to be present when patients and their families entered hospital, offering immediate support. That support generally included ensuring that patients and whānau understood the hospital procedures during and after initial assessments and throughout the patient's hospital journey to make them feel more comfortable in the environment. Another key role for Hunga Manaaki was to offer easy access to Māori therapeutic interventions if required. Several months after Hunga Manaaki began operating, some services noticed a significant drop in the number of formal complaints from patients and their families.[5] Hunga Manaaki services had a strong history of Māori goodwill and active participation, all geared towards improving Māori health outcomes.

From Amohaere's perspective, it seemed the experiences and needs of Māori patients in Auckland, Rotorua and Whakatāne were similar. It was the transfer of those identified cultural needs into a robust policy via the Kāhui Kaumātua of the local region that determined good practice.

In some ways, the processes of cultural sensitivity were made easier by having Māori co-ordinators who were already in place in the wards, albeit stretched to capacity. Education processes already set in place by locals who had seen Te Whānau Atawhai model in action also made the formal transition of Hunga Manaaki into hospital life easier. Amohaere's sister Phyllis worked in the Rotorua Hospital system, primarily in mental health. She had visited Starship years earlier to observe her sister's role as tumuaki. She soon saw the essential importance of biculturalism, Treaty education and cultural safety education and practice and was able to instigate similar education programmes in the mental health services associated with Rotorua Hospital. She had also opened a doorway for Amohaere's recommendations to make sense in this new environment.

Others like Ngāti Wāhiao kaumātua Uncle Rangitakatū Mihaka made a similar impact in the wards. He enjoyed visiting Māori patients in hospital so much that he had begun doing it regularly in the early 1990s as a volunteer.[6] He used to visit his relations in hospital and soon got talking to other patients, realising he knew the family or had some kin connection with them. Both Māori and Pākehā patients, especially the older ones, enjoyed speaking Māori to him and would often ask him to stay and continue talking with them. 'The kuia wouldn't let me go. They liked someone to talk to and they got lonely in the hospital. It's a healing process to our kuia to kōrero Māori with them. As soon as the patient saw me they were happy and I loved doing it,' he said.[7] Often patients' families acknowledged his caring contribution with koha of wild pork and other gifts of food.

Uncle Rangitakatū also remembered how many of the kaumātua could not communicate very well with the doctors, so he would speak Māori and interpret on their behalf. Initially, there were a couple of doctors who were not sure about his involvement, but after seeing how he could converse with patients and acquire information, they realised his worth. He says many of the staff at that time were interested in listening to him, asking for Māori words and questioning him about the Māori perspective. He also did karakia with the old people if they wanted it and, at times, would bless rooms after people had died. Patients would ask him about taking their own rongoā, and he would explain it to the doctors and get their okay.[8] This volunteer kaumātua Uncle Rangitakatū's caring actions represented everything that the elders of Te Whānau Atawhai, Amohaere and Auckland Hospital had recognised was an important and essential ministry for health consumers.

Lakes District Health Board's two hospital sites in Rotorua and Taupō provide care to over 100,000 people, covering an area of 9,570 square kilometres. The region they service stretches from Mourea in the north to Mangakino in the west down to Tūrangi in the south and across to Kāingaroa village in the east. It takes in the two main iwi groups of Te Arawa and Ngati Tūwharetoa.[9] These two tribal groups were hugely influential in advocating for Māori health workers, and key kaumātua worked tirelessly to help bring about a joint venture between Lakes District Health and Te Mana Hauora o Te Arawa (Te Arawa's recognised health authority).

In 1995, a new facility created by Lakeland Health and Te Mana Hauora o Te Arawa with assistance from Trust Bank Bay of Plenty brought about Paimārie, a whānau room project. It was the continuation of the Fraser Hostel facility, which was no longer in use, and was to accommodate caregivers and families during a family crisis.[10] Phyllis Tangitu was Te Hauora's representative in this venture.

It was a historical day on 16 August 1996. Te Arawa celebrated the beginning of a new era by signing a binding agreement with Lakeland Health for the delivery of health services appropriate to the local Māori community. The contract was the culmination of many years' work by the Crown Health Enterprise (CHE) and the local iwi and was based on Amohaere's cultural audit.

The signing by the CHE and Te Kāhui Hauora – the operational arm of Te Mana Hauora o Te Arawa, witnessed by ninety people at a ceremony at Rotorua Hospital, was a proud moment for local kaumātua. It was a recognition of how local Māori had sought greater involvement in health policy decisions and service delivery. And it was the fulfilment of a dream dating back to 1988[11] when Te Arawa Health Task Unit was set up under the umbrella of Te Arawa Māori Trust Board with the express objective of forming a comprehensive health plan for Te Arawa. In 1990, Te Arawa Health Authority became the mandated iwi authority to develop a health strategy and to work with the then operating area health boards. In 1992, all the Māori health-related bodies were merged into one Māori Health Authority – Te Mana Hauora o Te Arawa.[12] This was the entity that originally appointed Amohaere as iwi consultant to

Lakeland Health. And it was her report that was the foundation and the charter for the further development of the Hunga Manaaki entity.[13]

Under this 1996 joint agreement, Te Kāhui Hauora o Te Arawa was empowered to develop contracts for the health service within Te Arawa. Hunga Manaaki was contracted to practically deliver culturally appropriate care in the hospital wards and to boost the number of Māori working in health.[14] An additional joint tribal governance body was also formed to sit at a decision-making level. Te Roopu Hauora o Te Arawa (The Health Committee of Te Arawa) and Te Nohanga Kōtahitanga o Tūwharetoa (The Unified Seat of Tūwharetoa) joined together as an eldership of hapū representatives to sit as a governance body alongside Te Kāhui Hauora o Te Arawa. The elders who contributed to this eldership (1994–1997) were Te Pōroa Malcolm, Gunner Raharuhi, Bubbles Mihinui, Mary Tangitu, John Vercoe, Tūtānekai Kinita, Wihapi Winiata, Annie Paul, Kāwana Nēpia, Manny Kameta, Ella Bidois, Rangi Williams, Sam Hahunga, Taranaki Nuri, Marcia Tūhakaraina, Meihana Tūhakaraina, Whakapūmau Downes and others. This was another progressive move towards self-determination for Māori in the health arena.

All of this development could not have occurred without the support of key hospital staff who helped champion it under the umbrella of the Bicultural Action Team, or BAT as it was known. This team was driven by the desire to actively support the development of Hunga Manaaki and to promote its benefits to staff. Māori leaders guided the development of the Hunga Manaaki service with Lakes District Health Board Chief Executive Cathy Cooney, a professional nurse advisor and a member of the committee, negotiating details of the joint venture contract with Te Kāhui Hauora Trust during 1996.[15]

While they had initially considered bringing the Hunga Manaaki team on to staff, with advice, Cathy Cooney and the board decided to award the contract to Te Kāhui Hauora. This would mean the new team was employed by an agency that completely understood kaupapa Māori services. The contract committee was confident that as the operational arm of Te Mana Hauora o Te Arawa, Te Kāhui Hauora had excellent credibility and the required skills to make this joint venture contract work. The committee spent some months considering what roles Hunga Manaaki would play and the number of team members needed and built a business case for the financial requirements, working closely with Te Kāhui Hauora trustees throughout this process.

*

In the early days of Hunga Manaaki, there were very few referrals, largely due to the belief that people already did what its team members proposed to do. It was all too common for the cleaner to be asked to bless a room after a death. The cleaner would then go home and talk to a kaumātua to make sure he had carried the right tikanga. Now, contacts were to be set up with the chaplain or trained Hunga Manaaki staff to carry out these necessities.[16]

An early champion for the service was Lakes DHB Medical Director Johan Morreau. He reported that the Woman, Child and Family Service was one of the earlier services at Rotorua Hospital to receive the support of the Hunga Manaaki.[17] He believed there was a significant need for it, and he helped Hunga Manaaki team members to evolve their roles.[18] 'Support from health professionals working in the child health area was always strong. There's no question that Hunga Manaaki staff were hugely helpful, particularly as facilitators, dealing with some of our most difficult situations and helping to generate trust,' he wrote.[19] These situations largely involved Māori families experiencing significant stress in areas such as the Children's Unit, ICU (Intensive Care Unit) and ED (Emergency Department).[20]

Dr Morreau noted that there was clear recognition of the value in calling on Hunga Manaaki to facilitate family conferences and to support good family-based decision making. This approach helped smooth the way for decisions around issues such as withdrawing care and educating families around what was happening to their family member. He said another really important role for Hunga Manaaki was the ongoing education of non-Māori staff about dealing with issues involving Māori patients in a culturally appropriate way.[21]

Patients at times struggled to understand the information that they were receiving. Sometimes, Hunga Manaaki staff became involved in translating the English clinical instructions into Māori, but often it was about making the information more understandable for patients and their whānau to make hospital a less scary place for them. The team members also worked hard to help clinical staff understand the importance of whānau input and the spiritual components involved in helping people become well again.[22]

Implementing cultural safety into the system wasn't easy. Long-term Hunga Manaaki employee Michael Naera was involved in incidents where Hunga Manaaki staff had to make cultural calls against clinical recommendations. One whānau was asked to leave the ward because the patient, an elderly woman, was unable to rest. However, after the team members visited the family, they judged that the old lady really needed her whānau at that time. Shortly afterwards, she died, surrounded by her whānau rather than, as would have been the case, alone.[23]

At times when there were high profile deaths, Hunga Manaaki were called on to manage sections of the hospital. For example, the emergency department could be swamped with distraught whānau and huge numbers of people outside, making it difficult for normal hospital process to continue.[24]

Hunga Manaaki gradually made excellent relationships with pathologists, laboratory and mortuary assistants and the police.[25] Pathologists slowly became more accepting of a Māori view of death and of allowing bodies to be released on the day of death if a post-mortem was not needed.

Cathy Cooney commented that key clinicians were pivotal in their support and commitment to make the new service work. 'Hunga Manaaki was a radical development a decade ago,' she reported in 2007, 'but is now part of who we are as an organisation and part of what we do … the Hunga Manaaki service is now very much accepted as part of the multi-disciplinary team approach to patient care'.[26]

Amohaere's Iwi Consultancy Report had been the foundation of the development of Hunga Manaaki and a number of other initiatives.[27] (Leaping forward in time, it was with sadness Amohaere heard in June 2017 of the demise of Hunga Manaaki. The *New Zealand Herald* reported on the axing of Hunga Manaaki's services to Rotorua Hospital and that it was to be replaced by a Whānau Ora model with a wider community focus. Local members and supporters of Ngati Whakaue protested the actions of the Lake District Health Board and rallied at the hospital to support the reinstatement of Hunga Manaaki. An agreement was made to have further dialogue on this kaupapa).[28]

*

In 1997, Ngāti Awa kaumātua Charlie Vercoe and Eastern Bay District Health Board CEO Ron Dunham invited Amohaere to a community health hui in Whakatāne. Amohaere had known Ron from the days when he was general manager of Auckland Hospital. Tūhoe elder Hohepa Kereopa also attended this hui. Ron outlined the hospital's need to create and develop a Māori strategy to ensure the local district health board was delivering to this segment of its community. He also spoke about wanting to create an iwi consultant position as a helping hand to Hohepa in his position as a kaiāwhina (helper), overloaded with duties that were often outside the scope of his current brief.

'I didn't really know how Hohepa coped all these years with the workload he had on his shoulders. He and the Māori wardens he had commissioned had put a number of cultural tikanga in place, but there was no policy at senior management level to enforce these ways in general hospital practice,' Amohaere remembers.

At that hui, Ron approached Amohaere about returning to Whakatāne to work amongst her own Mataatua people. There were definite structural changes in the wind for the newly formed Eastbay Health. It was going to need careful thought and expertise as it entered a new phase of development, with a stronger commitment to local Māori health status and delivery of services for Māori.[29] Ron knew what was required but had no idea of the how. This would be a fortuitous opportunity for Amohaere to fulfil her dream of going home to her Ngāti Awa people.

The desire to return to her birthplace once again filled Amohaere with apprehension. She had endured a number of years of praise and criticism from her Te Arawa relations, but she knew that stepping into the Mataatua district would be a completely different story. Her role in Rotorua had been completed and could easily be left in the good hands of the people at Te Mana Hauora o Te Arawa. Weighing up all her options, and with the support of her whānau and tribal elders, Amohaere decided to take up her next challenge.

ELEVEN

Tangata Whenua Realities

In 1997 Amohaere agreed to return to Whakatāne to consult with iwi and undertake an audit of the cultural awareness of the Eastbay Health Crown Health Enterprise's (CHE) staff, patients and community.

Eastbay Health's region spread out from Ōtamarākau to Whangaparāoa in the Eastern Bay of Plenty. The Eastbay Health Board recognised that 45 percent of its client base was Māori and was committed to providing a better quality of service for them. To achieve this, Eastbay Health Manager Ron Dunham believed they needed to create a clear and definitive relationship with the local regional iwi.[1]

Amohaere's proposed consultation and review aimed primarily to strengthen and determine relationships with iwi, assess the current Eastbay health services for Māori and identify areas for improvement. The review was also to assess the attitude, knowledge and understanding of Eastbay staff in respect of the health service for Māori and identify what culturally related training was needed.[2]

At the helm of the consultation process, Amohaere expected many issues to arise. Stepping into this new role would be challenging. As a Ngāti Awa person who had not lived on her home soil for over thirty years, she knew she would have to find a way to fit back into the community mould. 'It's one thing having whakapapa links to a community but another to return as an unknown face hoping to find your position amongst the people again. They didn't know who I was; they hadn't really seen my face for many years. For me it was all about listening to what the people had to say.'

One of the first hurdles Amohaere faced was being compared to her son Pouroto (Nicholas) who had been living back in the Whakatāne region amongst Ngāti Awa for a number of years. Pouroto had a growing profile in the region and great knowledge of the Māori world. People automatically assumed Amohaere had the same calibre of Māori competence as her son. But this was certainly not the case.

Amohaere was formally welcomed home on to Umutahi Marae at Matatā. 'I was privileged to come back home to where I was born. It was also hard to come home to your own people. They have high expectations of you, and they were suspicious,' she told a news reporter at the time.[3] The suspicion was not just about her; it was also about the system she now represented that had failed Māori for many years. For too long, iwi were not part of the decision-making process.[4] That was something Amohaere was keen to set right. Nevertheless, at the pōwhiri for her own induction into this position, Ngāti Awa elders threw down a challenge to her employers. 'The proof,' they said, 'will be in the pudding.' In other words, 'Let's see what she can do.'

Based at Whakatāne Hospital, Amohaere formed the view that few of the staff and management had any rapport with the Māori community beyond that of the staff–client relationship. There was little rubbing of shoulders between management and the local tribal executives. Amohaere sensed the old suspicion of Māori towards hospitals was still alive and well.

Among the key Māori participants at the hospital were kaumātua Puti O'Brien and Wharekaihua Coates who sat on the hospital board. Both were related to Amohaere. There was also Tūhoe kaumātua Hohepa Kereopa, a recognised tohunga, and Makere Whakamoe. These were the first two kaiāwhina and had been with the hospital since 1989.[5] Hohepa had visited Amohaere previously to seek her advice about medical practice and cultural awareness. However, he now felt her presence at the hospital might usurp his mana. Amohaere reassured him that she could never carry out his role on the ground with local families: only he possessed the mana to work in that local field. As far as she was concerned, they had to work together; their roles were complementary, not opposing. With that clarified, Hohepa became instrumental in opening many doors for Amohaere and Eastbay Health to form relationships with many local iwi.

In her review of Eastbay Health's governance structure, Amohaere observed how silent the voice of Ngāti Awa was, considering the hospital was located within their tribal area. The hospital was built on land known as 'Ōtamakaukau o Pūkeko', which had originally belonged to Ngāi Tonu and Ngāti Pūkeko. She realised there was no contribution of any sort from Ngāti Awa as the mana whenua in the decision making around their own people's health. The board had regarded Hohepa's mana and advice as sufficient. When Amohaere asked Hohepa who the local Ngāti Awa kaumātua for the hospital were, 'Kare kau' ('There are none') was his answer. During the review process, Hohepa graciously resigned from his position to allow Ngāti Awa mana whenua to emerge.

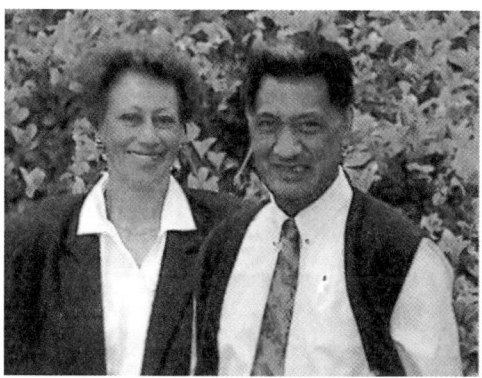

Amohaere meets with Hohepa Kereopa when she first arrives home to take up a position at Whakatāne Hospital in 1998.
COURTESY OF TE WHĀNAU O IRĀKEWA

A local Kaumātua Council of Mataatua elders was subsequently established to be a strong cultural arm for Eastbay Health and to advise Amohaere how to move amongst the tribes during her consultation process. This council was mandated by the board to move on their behalf. This was a milestone for Amohaere and the home people, who now had an authoritative body to represent them. Elders of the calibre of Wharekaihua Coates, Wiremu Maunsell, Bill Maxwell and others quickly came up with a communication plan to move into Murupara, Ruatahuna and throughout the region to make relationships.

'In my mind, the formation of a mandated Kāhui Kaumātua Council was the beginning of Ngāti Awa's decision-making power being validated over their own lands again and the future of their own health,' Amohaere says. 'There was a lot of talk at the time about rangatiratanga and what that really meant. It was a word bandied around, but most people were ignorant of what this thing called self-determination looked like, how it operated and its expression. Here was an opportunity for our people to determine and govern their own health needs.'

The occasion on which she felt Ngāti Awa stepped up to the mantle of claiming back their mana whenua and expressing their rangatiratanga with Eastbay Health was when Ngāti Awa elders came to bless the hospital and its grounds. A number of incidents had occurred on the site related to the processes of establishing the local Kāhui Kaumātua. Hospital cleaners told Amohaere about areas they believed needed urgent karakia or blessing. In the old Whakatāne buildings, staff would often hear a baby crying or see an old kaumātua standing in the corner. Other spirits were seen throughout the wards. Amohaere found unidentified human remains and foetuses stored in jars in the hospital basement that needed to be buried properly.

For Amohaere, this kind of environment created an unsafe space that exposed everyone – staff and patients – to a possible state of unwellness. Ascertaining whether the spiritual entities had been generated out of the history of the hospital itself or from an earlier time on the land was an issue that needed to be put to rest.

Having an understanding of and a relationship with the spiritual realm is imperative in this environment, Amohaere believes. Hospitals often employed staff chaplains, most of whom she feels have little knowledge of wairua and were not trained to handle wairua Māori situations. 'Quite frankly, in my experience, Pākehā are scared to bits of this spiritual world.' This was where local elders needed to be called in. It made sense, considering the hospital was built on Ngāti Pūkeko and Ngāti Awa lands, that it was their responsibility to settle these types of affairs.

Te Hau Tutua, Pouroto Ngaropo and Te Wharekaihua Willie Coates arrived at the hospital to perform the necessary karakia whakawātea (clearing incantations). Te Hau had always known this process was needed, but there had been no avenue previously for Ngāti Awa to settle it. With their arrival, some of the kaumātua realised Ngāti Awa had had little say about the hospital site and the activities associated with the health of their people. Amohaere saw this as a pivotal moment for the Kāhui Kaumātua in the region as they realised the mana whenua of Ngāti Awa at the hospital needed to be raised and recognised. 'Standing in the centre of the hospital as the karakia were recited to clear the old buildings of the past and to bless the site of the new hospital buildings was an important day for me personally. It was the day Māori values and spirituality were recognised by the local health system. I saw the tino rangatiratanga of the mana whenua established here at that very moment.'

In contrast to this, there were many who were suspicious and opposed to having Māori at a governance level. Others believed the hospital belonged to the

Pākehā, and Amohaere shouldn't be meddling in 'their' affairs. Some believed the elders were 'hell-raising' and bringing trouble with their karakia, while others felt discriminated against. Things were just getting 'too Māori' some voices shouted. It was all too familiar to Amohaere. Tender care and open sharing was needed to calm community fears and in particular those of the hospital staff.

'Building the open collective is hard work and takes a lot longer than people think. It cannot be simply cut and pasted from elsewhere; you have to get the sanction of the elders, and at the end of the day, with perseverance, it is a lot more satisfying,' Amohaere states.

Elders with connections to the other iwi travelled on the road with Amohaere and Ron Dunham to help open doors to the local communities. Kaumātua Charlie 'Te Nani' Vercoe, Peggy Wetini, Hohi Rangi and Pouroto all contacted their networks to carry this kaupapa to the communities. Travelling to key places to meet the tribal entities of the regions was not an easy task. Generally, the first twenty minutes on the many marae were filled with 'guns blazing' talk as the people poured out their historical grievances as major causative factors for their poor health. Seeing the health entity as a symbol of the government, the people would vent their anger. In Amohaere's experience the elders were key to handling this process. 'They knew how to gently answer the taunts of the people. There is always a test by our people when coming before them with issues that bring change. That's why it is essential to have elders move alongside the process. They easily detect the issues and offer wise solutions on the organisation's behalf.'

It was challenging for many of the elders walking alongside Amohaere in those days. They were overwhelmed by the vehement outpouring of threats and attacks against the system and the staff of the hospitals, but they overcame this with a listening ear and a genuine concern for the needs of the communities. It wasn't hard to see the health and social needs of the people. In many of the communities, housing was still inadequate, school buildings were cold and damp and people did not have transport. A service had to be specifically designed to meet their needs. In these cases, it was better to bring services to the people than expect them to come to the towns or cities.

Amohaere noticed how the women in these communities clearly took over the helm of responsibility for the health of the whānau and local people. For Amohaere, it was her grandmother, mother, her sister and other women like Aunty Puti O'Brien. The issues to do with karakia seemed to be the realm of men, yet men were often the main target of the regional health plan. As Amohaere saw it, Māori men were highly apathetic about their own health care.

*

The audit revealed that while the clinical management of care was 'sound', the cultural management of people was lacking. There was a clear need to improve the standard of delivery to Māori, who felt uncomfortable, particularly in inpatient services, owing to the lack of traditional practices such as blessing of beds in which other people had died. The food too was unfamiliar for Māori patients, particularly for the elderly. Māori staff needed support in dealing with bicultural aspects of health delivery. There was also a low number of Māori staff in influential positions. General staff were ignorant of bicultural and Treaty issues and how they impacted on Māori health. Amohaere identified a primary need to integrate Māori language with the overall treatment of Māori.[6]

Initiatives including biculturalism courses, the creation of a kaumātua council, providing a whānau house on site, training Māori staff and seeking additional employable staff[7] got underway. By September 1998, up to 200 (of 900) Eastbay staff had attended workshops, and sixteen Māori participants were nominated to attend a twenty-week management programme to help increase their understanding of the organisation and its structure.[8]

A major initiative resulting from the audit was the formation of two committees: Te Kupenga o Irākewa (the net of the prominent ancestor Irākewa); and a kaumātua advisory council, Te Kāhui Kaumātua Council (representatives of the twelve local tribes). These were set up under a formal memorandum of understanding with Eastbay Health.[9] Every member of both committees was to be nominated by their marae, hapū, rūnanga or iwi authority to represent their interests within Eastbay Health.[10]

Those who have sat on and contributed to these eldership councils since 1998 are Joe Mason, Te Nani Vercoe, Te Uru McGarvey, Paora Kruger, Rangipuke Tari, Bill Maxwell, Astrid Tāwhai, Mangu Clarke, Waireti Kīwara, Wī Parata Tawa, Puti O'Brien, Reuben Perenara, Katerina Waiari, Wiremu Maunsell, Rangi Williams, Taranaki Nuri, Ella Bidois, Whakapūmautanga Downes, Pouroto Ngaropo, Hawiki Ranapia, Rita Wordsworth, Dennis Waata Thomas, Hieke Tupe, Tahu Taia, Adelaide Waititi, Arapeta Te Rire, Mary Tangitu, Hohi Rangi, Mary Sykes, Wikita and Takaia Thomas, Marcia and Meihana Tuhakaraina, Andre Pateron, Miriama Gillies, Rangitukehu Paora, Sonny Rua, Sue Barton, Maraea Johns Turuwhenua, Rachel Kingi, Isaac Maereroa, Marcia Rakuraku and many others.

The Irākewa council's primary aim would be to help boost the number of Māori employees by being more involved in the process of writing employment descriptions, interviews and the selection process for Māori staff.[11] It was felt if more Māori faces were seen on staff, Māori patients would be more comfortable being treated by their own, and this, in turn, would assist better recovery.

Within a two-year period, eight positions were allocated, including a general manager and Māori staff. Amohaere was appointed as Pou Taratu Senior Manager Māori Health in 1998, under the direction of Pacific Health Whakatāne Hospital Manager, Karen Smith. Eventually, two positions designated as Māori health workers or pou kōkiri (advanced pillars) were allocated to this service. Amohaere's son Pouroto was employed as the project manager to administer Te Pou Kōkiri liaison service for the hospital. He worked within the mental health sector, the rehabilitation arena and in community health. Part of his role was to identify Māori needs and to create a strategically designed delivery service for them.

These placements saw the eventual establishment of Te Whānau o Irākewa: Māori Health Services Whakatāne in 2000, with both Te Kupenga o Irākewa and the Kāhui Kaumātua becoming a combined advisory board to Te Whānau o Irākewa Māori Health Services unit and personally accountable to Amohaere.

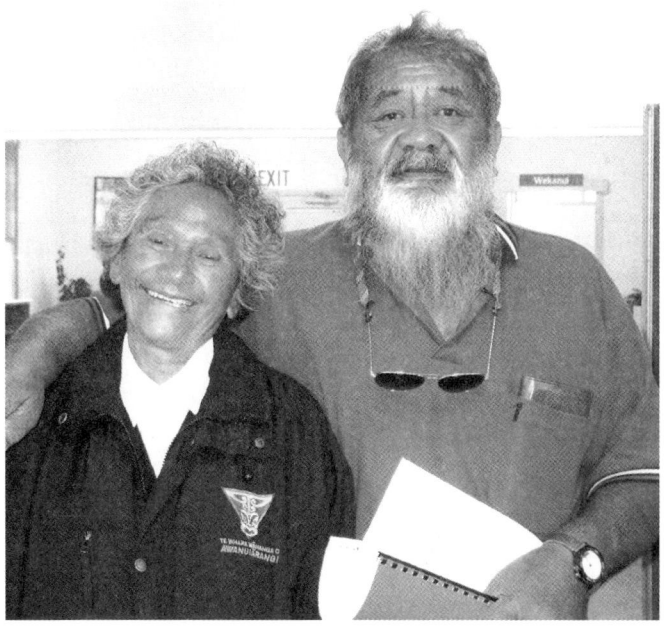

Te Whānau o Irākewa Kāhui Kaumatua Council elders
Katarina Waiari and Tāne Rakuraku.
COURTESY OF TE WHĀNAU O IRĀKEWA

*

The Eastbay Health consultation process got even more complex in 1999 with another change in the structure of the District Health Board. It was proposed that the Eastbay and Western Bay of Plenty health districts merge as Whakatāne Hospital had become financially unviable. Combining the two hospitals would keep services alive in Whakatāne. Māori clientele at Tauranga Hospital was 15 percent while Whakatāne had 45 percent.

Under this plan, Western Bay of Plenty Health and Eastbay Health would come under the new Bay of Plenty District Health Board. A new set of negotiations with iwi reaching as far west as Ngā Kurī a Whārei ki Tihirau from Bowentown to Whangaparāoa inland to Kaimai, Mamaku, and into the Urewera regions would be needed. For Amohaere, this meant expanding the timeframes for her team's consultancy work to enhance the relationships with eighteen tribes.

The advisory kaumātua suggested a team of elders accompany Amohaere and Ron Dunham, who was extremely supportive of kawa and tikanga, to the wider regions. They were unanimous in their decision to send Pouroto Ngaropo with the team because of his ability as an orator in the reo and his knowledge of tikanga. It meant travelling to over a hundred marae and consulting with Ngāi Te Rangi, Ngāti Pūkenga, Ngāti Ranginui, Waitaha, Tapuika, Ngāti Whakaue, Ngāti Rangitihi, Ngāti Whakahemo, Ngāti Mākino, Tūwharetoa ki Kawerau, Ngāti Awa, Tūhoe, Whakatōhea, Ngāti Manawa, Ngāti Whare, Ngāi Tai, Te Whānau a Te Ehutu and Te Whānau-a-Apanui. The team sought to appraise the tribes' specific health needs as well as get buy-in from the people to participate on a multi-tribal rūnanga (council) that would sit at a governance level alongside the health board.

This perseverence led to the Bay of Plenty District Health Board (BOPDHB) welcoming Te Rūnanga o Te Moananui o Toi (the Council of the Great Ocean of Toi), which represented the eighteen tribes, to sit at the table. As a multi-tribal rūnanga, it would represent the interests of whānau, hapū, iwi and 160 marae within the district health board region, which then had a population of 180,000. Fourteen percent lived in decile 10 areas, and one in four were Māori, and there were higher proportions of children and elderly than the New Zealand average.[12]

With these statistics it made sense to establish a Māori voice such as the Rūnanga o Te Moananui o Toi, to provide leadership and strategic direction to the BOPDHB at a governance level and to provide advice on matters pertaining to the impact of health and disability services for Māori. Both the Tauranga

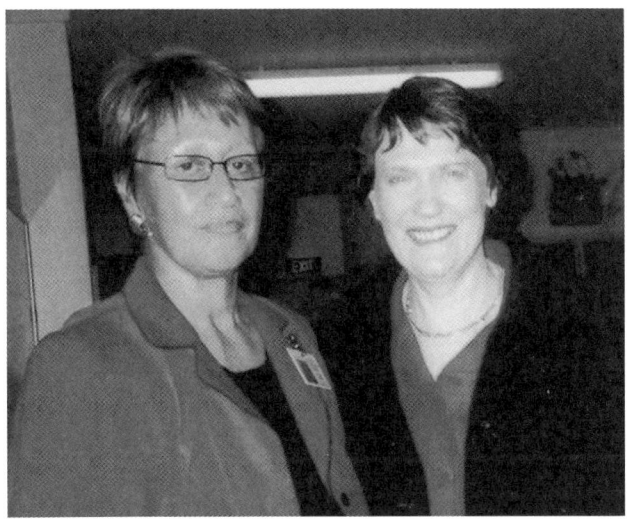

Amohaere with Prime Minister Helen Clark, who visited Whakatāne Hospital while on the campaign trail. It was the first time a pōwhiri (Māori welcome) had been performed at the hospital for a dignitary.
COURTESY OF TE WHĀNAU O IRĀKEWA

and Whakatāne hospitals now came under the BOPDHB, managed by Pacific Health Ltd, and included the territorial authorities of the Western Bay of Plenty, Tauranga, Whakatāne, Kawerau and Ōpōtiki.

Te Whānau o Irākewa Māori Health Services decided to operate under a blanket kaupapa Māori approach where Māori policy would apply to every client and staff member within Whakatāne Hospital. 'My view was to navigate through te ao Māori (the Māori world) and to weave the cultural fabric into the local health sector,' Amohaere says. The unit believed cultural safety was the responsibility of all health carers associated with this hospital, as opposed to the Tauranga Hospital kaupapa Māori strategy where they chose to establish Ward 2A in 2008 as a specific kaupapa Māori ward to meet the clinical and cultural needs of Māori patients. This was to be the only ward of its kind: an acute ward for medical, respiratory, diabetes and cardiac patients, providing a model of care based on whanaungatanga.[13]

At Whakatāne Hospital, Te Whānau o Irākewa was soon charged with the orientation of all hospital staff, including medical and management. The Tangata Whenua Cultural Safety policy, standards and procedures were issued and implemented in July 2000 but applied only to Pacific Health Ltd's Whakatāne Hospital and the Whakatāne region.[14] This policy recognised Whakatāne Hospital's commitment to the Treaty of Waitangi and to the delivery of service specifically to Māori. It also honoured its commitment to providing training opportunities. Staff would have individual responsibility to develop an understanding of culturally appropriate practice. The Māori manager was to be consulted over changes and accessed as a resource regarding service provision and quality issues as well as policy and procedure development. Pou kōkiri staff were to be available to all Māori clients in the wards and the community to support and advise whānau through the use of the reo and tikanga.

An addition to the cultural safety policy was 'The Blessing of the Room After a Patient Has Died', implemented under the 'Spiritual Care' section.[15] A blessing or cleansing would be carried out to commend the 'immaterial soul of the tūpāpaku' to his or her ancestral homeland and to cleanse the room and its linen and equipment so that a state of peace and tranquility would prevail.[16] The deceased's family had to be informed of the blessing and, along with staff, invited to participate if they wished. The celebrant, defined as a chaplain, te pou kōkiri, kaiāwhina, family member, registered staff, a family priest, tohunga or minita tautoko, had to perform the blessing. A room was not to be reallocated until the blessing had been completed.[17] Having these practices now embedded in policy was a far cry from the way health care had been administered to Amohaere and her family over forty years earlier.

*

As this cultural machinery began to grow teeth, it became increasingly clear to Amohaere how much she needed to fill the gaps in her own knowledge about the health sector, management, and the Māori world. In 2001, she signed up for a postgraduate Management in Health Studies programme at Waikato University. At the same time, she enrolled in a Diploma in Business Management and Māori Studies programme at Te Wānanga o Raukawa. 'I recognised that without the right qualifications, it would have been hard for me to have any further informed influence in the sector. I needed to have a broader picture of management.'

Despite her determination, trying to juggle travelling between Ōtaki and Hamilton to attend classes and write assignments, while still managing to walk the hospital wards, was extremely difficult. One surprising aspect of the Waikato programme was that there was no mention of any of the forward movement in Māori health, such as the work she'd been doing for years. There was nothing about the concepts of cultural safety, biculturalism or Dr Mason Durie's whare tapawhā health model. 'I couldn't understand why there was nothing in the papers dealing with these subjects. There seemed to be no acceptance or recognition in the education sector of any kind of Māori worldview in the health education arena.' Astonished and disappointed, Amohaere nevertheless completed her studies and received the qualifications she needed to progress personally in the management arena.

Between 2000 and 2003, Te Whānau o Irākewa progressed in a number of ways. In August 2002, the Eastbay Māori Health Services created its own facility, which was officially named Te Whānau o Irākewa and opened by the chairperson of the District Health Board, Mary Hackett (Mary Futter).[18] It was a poignant meeting for both Mary and Amohaere. Mary was the head nurse from Princess Mary Hospital days who, all those years ago, initiated the original push to include a Māori presence in the hospital system that saw Amohaere first employed. Now, here were the two of them joining together to launch an initiative that would extend the Māori voice and outreach into the Whakatāne region. In a newspaper article at the time, Amohaere said that the facility would give local iwi a choice of language and culture in all facets of treatment from emergency, intensive care, surgery, the children's ward and even maternity.[19]

During this time, there was also a push towards finding a local Māori framework to operate under. This was something Pouroto Ngaropo researched and developed into a proposal for the Māori Health Service, based on the needs and wishes of the Māori community. The title, *Ngā Pou Mana o Io (The Pillars of Io)*, was coined by Pouroto for a mode of practice based on a pre-colonial philosophy linked to the spiritual and traditional belief system of tangata whenua. Before the coming of the Pākehā, tangata whenua cultural norms included four core pillars that Pouroto identified as mana atua, mana tupuna, mana whenua and mana tangata. These more holistic cultural concepts, this research document claimed, would give the people optimum spiritual, cultural, mental, social and physical wellbeing.[20]

The research for this development was a combined effort between Māori Health Services and Māori Mental Health Services. It arose as the result of an internal audit within the four divisions of Mental Health Services and an external audit of the Mental Health Services by whānau, hapū, iwi, Māori health providers and providers of the Eastern Bay of Plenty region.[21] Their research showed how disconnected Māori were from their own spiritual beliefs, ancestral dimensions, land connections and family – a major indicator of tangata whenua unwellness.

This unwellness at all levels is described through the term haumate:

ha – the breath of life

u – instilled into you at conception

mate – unwellness at all levels, sickness, negative energy, unbalanced, death

The philosophy of *Ngā Pou Mana o Io* was developed as a pathway to move Māori from a state of haumate (unwellness) to a renewed position of hauora (wellbeing).[22] Hauora is detailed as:

ha – the breath of life

u – to be instilled into you at conception

o – the female element, the circle of life, no beginning and no end, the womb of creation, nourishment

ra – the male element, light, warmth, energy, nourishment, sustenance, growth, wellness at all levels

A brief summary of *Ngā Pou Mana o Io* is outlined below.

Mana Atua

- Recognises the spiritual values, beliefs and practices of whānau, hapū and iwi, waka and Māori communities
- Recognises the importance of the tohunga, kaumātua or any spiritual leaders in the ao Māori
- Recognises that all Māori have a spiritual origin that contributes to their holistic wellness

Mana Tupuna

This refers to the ancestral linkages of a person to their roots, to their blood ties and to their ancestral beginnings. A person who does not know who they are, is considered a lost soul. Having this second pillar enables Tangata Whenua to stand with pride, confidence, self-esteem and dignity.

- Recognising that whānau, hapū, iwi and waka have their own unique identity and autonomy
- When culturally relevant, allowing tangata whenua to implement their own cultural norms

Mana Whenua

This is the power associated with knowing the place of origin of your ancestors, despite those lands possibly being out of whānau, hapū and iwi hands.[23] This pillar recognises the connection to your place of identity.

- Recognisng that whānau, hapū, iwi, waka and Māori communities are the kaitiaki of their whenua, tūrangawaewae and wāhi tapu

- Contacting the right iwi in relation to environmental issues that impact on the health of whānau, hapū and iwi

Mana Tangata
- A person is born with the gifts of their ancestors through the lineage of their parents. Mana tangata is your connection to the descent group you belong to. This fourth pillar reinforces the importance of having the support of your whānau, hapū/marae, iwi and waka.
- Recognition of tangata whenua aspirations and their own communication systems
- One's own authority, quality, attributes
- Capacity for self-governance
- Tribal leadership and for Māori issues, whānau, hapū, and iwi having power of veto in discussing matters that will impact on their life ethos (See appendix 1 for further details.)

These four pillars contribute to the four dimensions of health from a holistic perspective. Further to this, it was proposed that te reo (the Māori language) and tikanga (values and beliefs) would be the vehicle of delivery of service to the Māori people. Another overarching principle in this model was to give Māori whānau, hapū, iwi, waka and Māori communities the time and opportunity to define, decide and protect their cultural interests for themselves and their families.[24]

After presenting this model to whānau, hapū and iwi within the western and eastern Bay of Plenty and to the hospital management, Ministry of Health, Mental Health and Māori Health services, it was agreed *Ngā Pou Mana o Io* could assist with identifying the indicators of tangata whenua health and wellbeing. Through the Māori Health Rūnanga representing eighteen iwi of the region, *Ngā Pou Mana o Io* was accepted in principle as the philosophy to ascertain tangata whenua determinants of health.[25]

During one presentation to local elders, Anglican church leader, Bishop Whakahuihui Vercoe stood up and commented strongly, 'I'm pronouncing my unwellness.' This was a validation for the ancient way, a pathway many of the elders present had not associated as being so deep in the context of health. Each of the elders followed Bishop Vercoe's lead and stood to celebrate this model as the way they would like to see the Māori Health Service in Whakatāne move forward.[26]

The four pillars were adopted by Te Whānau o Irākewa Māori Health Services as the principle guidelines for the implementation of Cultural Safety.[27] 'For me, there was a high level of excitement and expectation as our reo and tikanga were now validated as a component of health and care. The implementation of this model was new for people, and there were those who accepted it and many who resisted its style of delivery, especially in te reo Māori.' Amohaere wasn't surprised at the opposition, but she was insistent that the hospital in this region, which has a large Māori population and the second highest rate of Māori language speakers in the country, should offer the delivery of its service in the language of the people.

'The reo as a healing agent was not necessarily accepted by many, including by some of the tribal groups.' People would ask Amohaere why she was so passionate about the language. 'Because I know what it is to not have the reo and to not understand what is going on. I didn't have the full picture of my own Māori world,' she would answer.

Amohaere is a strong believer that speaking the reo and knowing how to stand and mihi validates one's connection to the patients and Māori families. 'I never want my own mokopuna to go through the pain and anxiety of not having the choice to access health services either in a Māori way or a non-Māori way. They must have the right to choose because the service actually exists now to have that choice.'

Implementing *Ngā Pou Mana o Io* meant creating a whole new set of standards, competencies, performance appraisals and training curricula. With cultural safety training initiatives devised for Toi Te Ora Community Health and Disability Services, Pacific Health sought to develop each participant's understanding and knowledge base of cultural custom, ritual, meanings and understandings pertaining to cultural safety practices. It was believed this would empower participants to be more culturally aware and competent when dealing with tangata whenua.[28] Understanding the Tangata Whenua Cultural Safety policy and Māori health status and being introduced to *Ngā Pou Mana o Io* became essential subjects in this training. So too was knowing the issues around the reo, its pronunciation, its power to communicate and its capacity as a healing agent. Traditional cultural concepts of tikanga, wairua, tapu, noa, mana, hauora, ihi, wehi, wana, wahine, ūkaipō, rāhui, iriiri and mauri were key subjects in the training manual. Becoming familiar with and applying these concepts in customer services as well as in the processes of death, the removal and return of body parts and the burial of the placenta were essential for participants if they were to truly engage with Māori.[29]

As it grew its capacity in terms of people and cultural competency, Te Whānau o Irākewa continued to consult with its iwi partners to meet the needs of the communities and the staff it served. The recognition of the Treaty of Waitangi and the tenets of partnership, participation and protection in the New Zealand Public Health and Disability Act 2000[30], the Bay of Plenty District Health Board charter and the Pacific Health (Whakatāne Hospital) policy gave Amohaere and Te Whānau o Irākewa a strong foundation to actively continue evolving. Partnership, participation and protection were identified by BOPDHB as Treaty principles in Māori health and were developed into a framework as a 'tool to operationalise the Treaty of Waitangi obligations'.[31]

In the board's 2004 document *He Ritenga*, partnership was defined as working together with whānau, hapū, iwi and Māori communities to develop strategies for Māori health gain and appropriate health and disability services. Participation meant involving Māori at all levels of the organisation in planning, development and delivery of health and disability services, while protection was about ensuring that Māori enjoy the same level of health as non-Māori and safeguarding Māori cultural concepts, values and practices.[32]

Amohaere believes that applying these tenets to management created something of a truly integrated health service where Māori values and spirituality were accepted in all aspects – from governance to delivery of services. This provided support and validation for the BOPDHB's strategic aim to achieve its key Māori health outcome: 'Healthy Māori'.[33]

In 2010, Amohaere was appointed Director Regional Māori Health Services. The selection panel felt that, aside from her curriculum vitae and credentials, it was Amohaere's continued commitment to walking the hospital wards to tend to the needs of patients that gave her the edge in being chosen for this role. Amohaere had a heart for the clients and the nous to work at every level of the hospital system.

TWELVE

Titiro Whakamua: Looking Forward

Nowadays, Amohaere lives with her immediate family at Awakaponga on Iramoko Marae, the home base for the Ngāti Awa hapū Te Tāwera. This marae stands on the tribal land known as Whāriki-te-toki. Since her move back to the Whakatāne region, Amohaere has been an avid participant in the tribal and community politics of the Ngāti Awa haukāinga. Her life's journey has come full circle: from a rural upbringing at Ōtākiri in a multigenerational whānau setting, then to bringing up her own family and working in an urban cityscape void of any real cultural lifestyle, and later returning home to become firmly established in the place of her true identity.

'A strong connection back to the haukāinga and to my whakapapa has been essential to my own personal wellness. It's only in the latter part of my life I have thought like this, as the heightened awareness of my own cultural understanding grew. I already knew I was lost when I lived in the city. There was an inner longing for wholeness, to know who I was and to understand my own Māoritanga. For me, where there is no wairua connection, unwellness reigns.'

The phenomenon of returning home to the papakāinga for whānau who shifted to the city years ago for work and education seems to be a common life-course journey for many Māori in their formative years. This was indeed true for Amohaere and her whānau. Even her husband, Sam, followed suit, returning home to the family marae to be with whānau in his final years. Amohaere was happy and relieved for their family's sake that Sam returned home – they had been separated for many years but never divorced. Sam eventually passed away but not before apologising to his sons for his past ways. While there may still be many things unspoken between family members, this was most certainly a healing moment for Amohaere and her sons. She has always believed change comes through honest truth telling, and it is never too late to make amends.

In her capacity as Regional Director Māori Health, Amohaere was responsible for managing Māori health services for both Tauranga (349 beds) and Whakatāne (110 beds) hospitals, while still walking the wards and teaching staff how to culturally care for the needs of Māori patients. For Amohaere, reaching this position in the workforce was never an easy road to walk. Since her entry into the hospital system in 1987, she was challenged by numerous obstacles, both personally and professionally. However, these complications enabled Amohaere to confront her own inadequacies and to conquer her own lack of confidence.

'Sometimes I felt like I was being forcefully pushed off this path. It was almost too hard,' she reflects. 'It was the encouragement of the elders that made me stay.' This support, along with her strong motivation to see Māori culture and people valued by the hospital system, saw Amohaere persist beyond her personal pain barrier to continue in the field.

She grew stronger in her conviction to see the health needs of the Māori community met and her own people take up the mantle of partnering with hospital management and making decisions for their own health. With the implementation of *Ngā Pou Mana o Io* within Te Whānau o Irākewa and later *He Pou Oranga Tangata Whenua, Tangata Whenua Determinants of Health Framework* (2007)[1], developed by Te Rūnanga Hauora o Te Moananui a Toi and the Bay of Plenty District Health Board, Amohaere felt Māori health principles that truly reflected tangata whenua realities were finally being recognised. For Amohaere, this was the fulfilment of a long-term vision.

'I wanted Māori to know they had an entitlement to a level of governance over their own health. To achieve this, they needed to be inside the tent not outside in the cold. Our people need to be participants of the solution process for a better health system, not just always being the clients or victims of that system. It's essential our people are involved at every level of the health spectrum if our voice is to be heard and our culture valued. It's not a time to be silent or to simply just accommodate old ways that are irrelevant to the lives of our mokopuna. We must be willing participants now for their sakes.'

Amohaere's ultimate goal has been to see hospitals take responsibility for cultural safety as a standard health practice and not just a Māori practice. 'For it to work, it had to be a whole systems approach where everybody, including staff, clinicians and managers, would take responsibility to administer both clinical and culturally appropriate care for the safety of all patients and their families.'

In reviewing the progress of this goal within her own arena of influence, Amohaere was elated to share with senior management one incident that demonstrated a real advancement of attitude and cultural action.

Staff from the Intensive Care Unit (ICU) at Whakatāne Hospital decided, of their own volition, to initiate a cultural practice to resolve a serious situation surrounding a patient's tragic circumstances. A severe car accident had seen a young woman, her mother and two children rushed into emergency. The two babies did not survive the accident, while the young woman and her mother were both in a terrible state in intensive care. Amohaere and Pouroto met with whānau who gathered in force at the hospital. The family elders were pleased to see them on site to ensure the correct tikanga was carried out in this situation. After medical checks were completed, Amohaere and one of the nurses carefully dressed the babies before presenting them back to the children's father and the wider whānau. 'It was truly devastating,' Amohaere recalls.

Nursing staff in the ICU were deeply saddened by the affair, knowing full well that the mother and the grandmother would not be able to mourn the babies' deaths or attend the imminent funerals. Everyone realised that the mother and grandmother would never see or hold the children again. So they initiated a move to seek the consent of all the patients and staff in the ward to bring the two infants' bodies in to lie next to their mother. They would hold the tangihanga in the ward for a day. As far as Amohaere knew, this was unheard of in this hospital.

In seeking an answer to their request, the staff were careful to cater for everyone's needs. There were no complaints by any staff or patients in the ward, and all were in agreement to allow the tangi to occur on site. So prior to being released to the undertaker, the two babies were carried in bassinets into the ward and gently set down beside their mother. It was a hugely emotional scene. Streams of people entered the ward to openly mourn, wail, pay tribute and offer their condolences in a traditional way. That day, staff and patients became part of the tangata whenua reality of mourning for the dead and openly expressing sympathy for the living. 'It was all so surreal,' Amohaere remembers.

Later, the children's family returned to thank everyone involved in making the tangihanga happen in the intensive care ward. 'The family did not have the words to express their thanks to the hospital,' Amohaere remembers. These were exceptional circumstances not seen by Amohaere in her career. She saw this situation as a milestone in the history of this hospital.

More than that, this event brought back painful memories for Amohaere as she was reminded of the days when she and her mother were unable to mourn the deaths of their own babies who had died in hospital. They both missed their own babies' funerals due to archaic hospital rules and circumstances totally out of their own control.

Amohaere honoured the fact that hospital staff had finally taken the initiative to take responsibility, not only for the safe clinical care of the people, but to step out of the box to administer unfamiliar but correct cultural practice. It signalled real progress. Here, two worlds came together for the full wellbeing of Māori and people in general. For Amohaere this was real bicultural health care in action. It was a satisfying moment seeing the culmination of years of hard work by so many people coming to fruition at this point.

'Oh, how the times have certainly changed! The sensitivity of attitudinal change towards Māori is a measure of what we are as a hospital, what we do and how we practise. The veneer held between New Zealand Pākehā and Māori is slowly but surely thinning and for me personally.'

Despite the enormous amount of work accomplished in the cultural safety arena, Amohaere is cautious as she reflects on how much work there is still to do. With the constant turnover of staff, doctors and nurses, the continued orientation of hospital staff into this way of practice is even more essential for the maintenance of cultural care. There is no room for sitting on our laurels, content with our achievements and not continuing with efforts for review and change, Amohaere contends.

Surveying the current status of Māori health, one of her primary concerns is the lack of health literacy amongst Māori. 'We need to be involved in educating our people in the area of health literacy. It is central to our overall wellness.'

Recent commentaries in a number of contemporary reports suggest a higher level of health literacy is needed for Māori to maintain their own wellness.[2] Health literacy is broadly defined as a person's ability to obtain, process and understand basic health information and services in order to make informed and appropriate health decisions.[3] More specifically, it is also the 'skills people need to find their way to the right place in the hospital, fill out medical and insurance forms, and communicate with their health providers'.[4] Māori across the labour-force spectrum and income quintiles, whether living as rural or urban dwellers, all have lower health literacy than non-Māori.[5]

Following through with medications and sticking to appointments are essential for Māori patients. Amohaere remembers how specific clinics booked for a hundred people would only see seventy arrive and the remainder would be identified as DNA (did not arrive).

'In Whakatāne, the rate of DNAs for health clinics was 50 percent. Encouraging better health compliance where our people attend tests and seminars for their own health is imperative,' Amohaere insists.

Cervical cancer smear tests are never comfortable for women, and more so for Māori women, who would not actively seek out the tests. In response to this, Amohaere would go out to the people, share with the women, then hold their hands as they were ushered into a comfortable environment to be tested.

Men's health is another big concern for Amohaere. 'Māori men are more apathetic about their own personal health. For example, those who suffer from gout are recommended to take specific tablets often for the rest of their lives to ward off the painful ailment. Many take the tablets until their gout symptoms disappear in the immediate timeframe, but this does not necessarily heal the overall illness.'

'On one occasion I remember seeing four Māori men in hospital aged between thirty and fifty years old. One of the men asked me if my husband drank; he insisted he might talk to him about the effects of alcohol.' Before Amohaere could reply, the man told her how alcohol was the reason all four of them were in hospital. All of them were dying he told her. All of those men eventually passed away from renal failure due to alcohol. 'In my upbringing, we never had alcohol. I never saw this state of illness till after I was married. Then I'd see drinking binges everywhere, including on the marae and at tangihanga – not just for three days but for a week at a time. So often this would lead to family violence.' After witnessing the devastating effects of alcohol on men, women and whānau, Amohaere advocates a no alcohol policy for families nowadays. 'I want to see our men well and see our hospitals closed; that would be my ultimate dream.'

Amohaere is adamant Māori language and tikanga are a major component in the definition of Māori wellness. 'It's part of what it means being Māori and being well. With the growth of te reo Māori speakers in the kōhanga and kura kaupapa world, this has meant we too as an organisation need to be more competent in the language if we are to offer equitable services to our people. Many kura kaupapa will only accept Māori-language-speaking doctors and health providers to their schools these days. That is their prerogative, and we must respect that.' She sees this as crucial to ensuring mokopuna Māori are not deprived of who they are as Māori. 'I wanted to create an environment that fosters Māori language and tikanga as I know what it feels like to be insecure without the reo and absent of culture as part of my identity and my wellbeing.'

Rapid changes in technology have also greatly influenced hospital and medical processes, extending even to the place of patient–doctor engagement. Phone calls and video conferencing have become an inevitable technical necessity, saving time where distance is an issue. For families living on the eastern Bay of Plenty coastline from Ōpōtiki to Tihirau, these facilities allow fast, efficient and immediate long-distance engagement between patients, doctors and clinicians. Amohaere advocates moving with the times, but she is cautious of the dehumanising factor attached to technology. It can be a barrier for Māori of her generation, some of whom have conveyed to her that they regard this process as not being tika.

'Meeting via electronic media makes it hard to create a genuine rapport between unknown faces or to carry out the process of kawa and tikanga in a meaningful way. From a cultural standpoint, kanohi ki te kanohi is still the preferred mode by which many of our people live.'

*

Amohaere's contribution to the progressive developments in Māori health was formally recognised at a celebration ceremony on 7 December 2012.[6] She was bestowed with the title of Distinguished Fellow – Māori Health Sciences (Nursing) by Te Whare Wānanga o Awanuiārangi indigenous university at Whakatāne. This was in recognition of the many outstanding contributions made by Judith Amohaere Tangitu towards developments in Māori health. Amohaere was awarded this honour alongside her cousin Sir Wira Gardiner, who received an honorary doctorate, and Te Onehou Phillis, who was posthumously awarded an honorary doctorate.[7]

Amohaere's citation was presented and signed by Distinguished Professor Sir Sidney Mead (Hirini Moko Mead), Chairman of Te Whare Wānanga o Awanuiārangi, and Distinguished Professor Graham Hingangaroa Smith, Chief Executive Officer of Te Whare Wānanga o Awanuiārangi.[8] The citation reads:

> This is to affirm the conferment of the title of Distinguished Fellow – Māori Health Sciences (Nursing) by Te Whare Wānanga o Awanuiārangi: indigenous university. It recognises the many outstanding contributions made by Judith Amohaere Tangitu towards developments in Māori Health. Amohaere was born in Whakatāne

and raised in Ōtākiri, a rural settlement in the Eastern Bay of Plenty. Her iwi affiliations are Ngāti Awa, Ngāti Pikiao, Ngāti Ranginui, Ngāi Te Rangi and Ngāti Maniapoto. For many years she has been a strong supporter on a number of tribal marae including Umutahi and Iramoko. Her career began in the 1960s as a nurse aide at Kawerau Maternity Hospital. After raising her family, she took up a position in 1987 at the Princess Mary Children's Hospital in Auckland, holding one of the first Māori posts in a mainstream health organisation in New Zealand. Key objectives of that position included creating a safe environment for urihaumate and their whānau, ensuring the health professionals practised in a manner appropriate for Māori, advocating for children and their whānau to ensure whānau involvement in care and treatment, providing education and developing wider community as well as iwi and hapū relationships. These same objectives remain a focus of her work today as the Regional Director of Regional Māori Health Services, Hauora a Toi, Bay of Plenty District Health Board. The involvement of Amohaere over many years in the field of Māori Health has included the development of Māori Health Services Te Whānau Atawhai; the establishment of Te Whānau Atawhai Kāhui Kaumātua Council; the development and support of Treaty of Waitangi Programmes; Introduction of Cultural Competencies for Nurses at Carrington Polytechnic, Manukau Institute of Technology and Auckland Institute of Technology; the provision of Cultural Competencies Programme for Clinical Placement Students at Auckland Hospital; as a Surveyor with the New Zealand Council of Healthcare Standards specific to Māori health needs; and her extensive participation over the years with the programmes at Starship Children's Hospital. In recognition of her outstanding contribution to Māori health development and support for Te Whare Wānanga o Awanuiārangi the title of Distinguished Fellow – Māori Health Sciences (Nursing) is bestowed upon Judith Amohaere Tangitu by Te Whare Wānanga o Awanuiārangi: Indigenous University.

The award stands not only as a tribute to Amohaere and her influence in the mainstream hospital system in Auckland, Rotorua and Whakatāne but also as a fitting recognition by her own iwi of her achievements in acknowledgement of her service to the people.

*

More recently in early 2018, Amohaere reluctantly accepted an enhanced retirement package after many years pushing for equity and partnership between Māori and hospital management and walking the wards of hospitals caring for and monitoring the cultural needs of Māori patients.

Looking back on her career, Amohaere identifies the hero she modelled her style of leadership and management on was not a person but the concept of whanaungatanga – the maintenance of kin and non-kin relationships and the expression of associated obligations towards each other. Maintaining the family unit in a state of whanaungatanga has always been a primary motivation for Amohaere in her outlook for Māori health and wellbeing. It was derived from her own childhood memories of living in a world where whanaungatanga was paramount.

'The whanaungatanga expressed in the family home was a reflection of the wider community. In those days, we all respected the boundaries within that whanaungatanga, set down by the elders. There was never any question of who did what and what had to occur at any given moment. The boundaries were a safeguard within our home relationships and between our wider kin, but somehow it kept us in the centre of belonging. It depended on everyone keeping their mutual obligations towards each other in check. We need this today, especially in the relationships between patients, staff and families.'

Whanaungatanga became an essential mode of practice in Amohaere's style of management; its Māori origin and inclusive nature appealed to her. 'It came naturally,' she says. 'Years ago it was adopted as a way of leadership, exemplified by Te Kāhui Kaumātua elders of Te Whānau Atawhai. We applied the principles of whanaungatanga alongside awhi, manaaki, and atawhai into mainstream, which was the basis for relationship with urihaumate, staff and leadership. It was no easy task to achieve.'

Her leadership style has always been to do rather than to dictate. 'It's inclusive not exclusive and has been based on wide consultation with elders before any action was to be carried out.' However, as she remarks, 'At the end of the day, the final call was always thrown back to me to manage and implement their decisions.'

Amohaere believes what she has learned over the years is the power of intentional expression of identity as a requirement of health and wellbeing. 'I realised way back in the 1980s we did not value our own identity, and I saw the effect of this on our own wellness. We have tolerated others' dominating racist attitudes over us.' This realisation has been a driving force in Amohaere's vision, which is to see Māori self-determination in health. This is something that has been realised to a degree through the formation of tribal councils participating at management, policy and decision-making levels within the system, determining the cultural tikanga for their own people's health needs.

'Māori can survive mainstream!' Amohaere insists. 'We must create a scenario where the hospital actually becomes defunct or redundant because the health of the people is good, where Māori people grow in their own health so they will not need the hospital system at all. Until that time, whether we like it or not, clinical and cultural care must walk together for the sake of wellbeing.'

This dual progression of clinical and cultural care is epitomised in the proverb 'Rapua te huarahi whānui hei ara whakapiri i ngā iwi e rua i runga i te whakaaro kōtahi' ('Seek the broad highway that will unite the two peoples towards the common goal'), which Amohaere has always advocated throughout her career within mainstream. However, looking back, Amohaere recognises there is a difficulty in maintaining this trajectory within mainstream – its name is complacency.

Complacency will stagnate growth, destroy vision, stifle creativity and cause an aversion to risk taking. Amohaere is adamant the only way to break free from the bonds of complacency is to continually challenge the status quo. This means confronting ourselves, our personal prejudices and racial discrimination in the system.

One particular area Amohaere admits will need rigorous attention in the very near future is successive Māori leadership. This revelation occurred to her in 2017 while spending months sleeping in the intensive care ward nursing and supporting her son Christian who was suffering from cancer. Her observation of staff treatment of her son and other Māori patients was disappointing and disheartening.

'It appeared to me, the treatment and communication towards a patient who is unwell as opposed to a dying patient was different. Staff treated difficult and dying patients, my son included, with a lack of full concern and attention, often not recognising that difficult patients' issues could be alleviated simply by keeping the urihaumate comfortable and managing their pain levels,' she says. 'Good pain management allows the patient to communicate more easily and to be part of what is happening around them.'

She also observed the communication styles between doctors, nurses and patients was not safe at all. 'Instead of asking the patient or the family what their thoughts would be in a possible fatal situation, doctors would launch into in-depth descriptions of the breakdown of the body leading to death. This was totally inappropriate. There was sometimes little care taken in the delivery of messages by staff, to the point that Māori patients did not feel safe. They didn't want to hear how death occurs because it was fearful. Our people still say nothing in these situations and don't want to complain. They're scared they may have to return to the hospital again only to be treated by the same staff, who may not treat them properly. So they say nothing.'[9]

Caring for her son right up until his passing and witnessing how he was treated, Amohaere wondered, for the tiniest of moments, whether all the years of cultural safety intervention were really worth it or if she had been complacent. She wondered how this kind of attitude and treatment could still occur with all the cultural safety training in place or whether this kind of attitude was due to the patients just being Māori.

'My long-term expectations of the current system changed as I realised there is still so much more work to do. We must not relax. While I have worked in this system for this length of time, your feelings of vulnerability as a mother and a family member can only be described if you've experienced it.' It is evident too that the treatment of the elderly by nurses and doctors in the wards requires more cultural sensitivity.

Amohaere is certain more education, more monitoring and more sharing of patients' experiences is needed to inform the way culturally safe treatment is administered and delivered. 'This is ultimately a leadership issue that needs rectifying. More Māori leaders need to be raised up to positions across the full spectrum of the health system.'

In reviewing all the education, training and orientation taught over the years in the fields of cultural safety, biculturalism and the Treaty of Waitangi, Amohaere came to the realisation that a correction in strategy had to occur for this education to be more effective. 'There is no education programme for current leadership that includes a higher level of Te Ao Māori learning as well as offering opportunities for Māori to be educated into more influential positions within an organisation's leadership strategy'.[10] She strongly believes progressive Māori leadership and succession in the health field should be a high priority to achieve the Bay of Plenty District Health Board aim of Māori health – achieving equity.[11]

Just prior to her retirement, Amohaere sought to devise a programme to enhance non-Māori leaders' cultural intelligence and to plan specific strategies to enable them to support Māori leadership ambitions. It was a programme based on He Awa Whiria – Braided Rivers approach developed by Professor Angus Hikairo Macfarlane, which draws on the analogy of parallel streams of thought flowing from western science and kaupapa Māori to create a melting pot of complex ideas where true partnership and effective development could emerge.[12] Amohaere sought to apply this approach to a newly developed leadership programme to bring kaupapa Māori and western science together so that each could inform, develop and be used to evaluate the other, encouraging 'partnership, co-operation and convergence between the two'.[13]

For Amohaere, this approach would require a proactive stance from those in positions of influence and responsibility. Managers and leaders would need to advance their competence by being strongly engaged in Tiriti-based cultural intelligence and partnership to enhance Māori health gain, ensure cultural safety and strategise Māori staff leadership succession.[14] 'It would be an opportunity to embed the principles of Te Tiriti o Waitangi and He Pou Oranga Tangata Whenua into all management and leadership practice,' she says. Ensuring Māori leadership in the Bay of Plenty District Health Board, she declares, must be maintained and sustained.

*

Amohaere's parting statement at this time of her life is apt and fitting.

'I wanted to set a benchmark of standards that would become the norm in mainstream and must be maintained by the next generation. This was never a job to me. It was a commitment to my people.'

She continues, 'I hope the people will sustain the idea of keeping the needs of patients at the forefront, to do what needs to be done from their perspective, not ours. Our role has been to intervene with patients before clinical care is administered. If we could reduce a bad hospital experience, then this becomes the measure of the validity of the service. Illnesses and disparity are preventable these days, and, in theory, we should be getting well.'

APPENDIX 1

Chapter Eleven

Ngā Pou Mana o Io (The Pillars of Io)

Mana Atua

This is the spiritual connection of tangata whenua to its highest sources of wellbeing, which includes Karakia Tūturu Māori. A person without the knowledge and understanding of their spiritual essence becomes a 'wairua manakore' or a disconnected soul. Mana Atua seeks to connect people to the source of their spiritual origins and in this case it begins with Io. According to Pouroto, 'I' in Io translates to mean 'Ihi', that is the vitality force, the sacred seed of creation, the male element. The 'O' in Io translates to mean 'Oho' to be awake, alert, aroused, the circle of life that has no beginning and no end. The female womb of creation. Io also means: balance, equality, equilibrium, a state of being at peace. The full explanation of Ngā Pou Mana o Io traces the epochs of time from Io to the main seven progeny of Ranginui and Papatūānuku, being Tāne, Tūmatauenga, Rongomātane, Haumietiketike, Tāwhirimātea, Tangaroa and Whiro.

APPENDIX 2: PHOTOGRAPHS

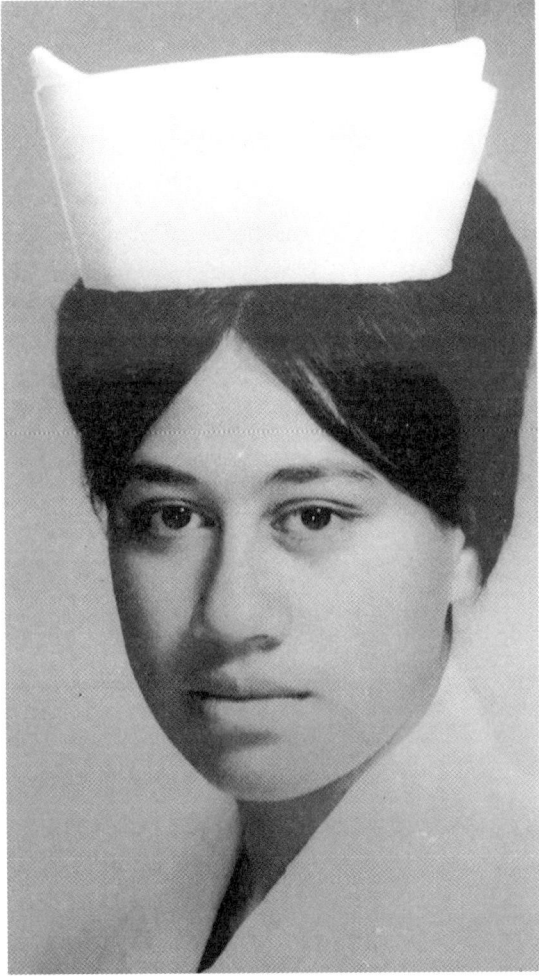

A young Judith Amohaere Tangitu as a trainee nurse at Whakatāne Hospital.
COURTESY OF AMOHAERE TANGITU

BRINGING CULTURE INTO CARE

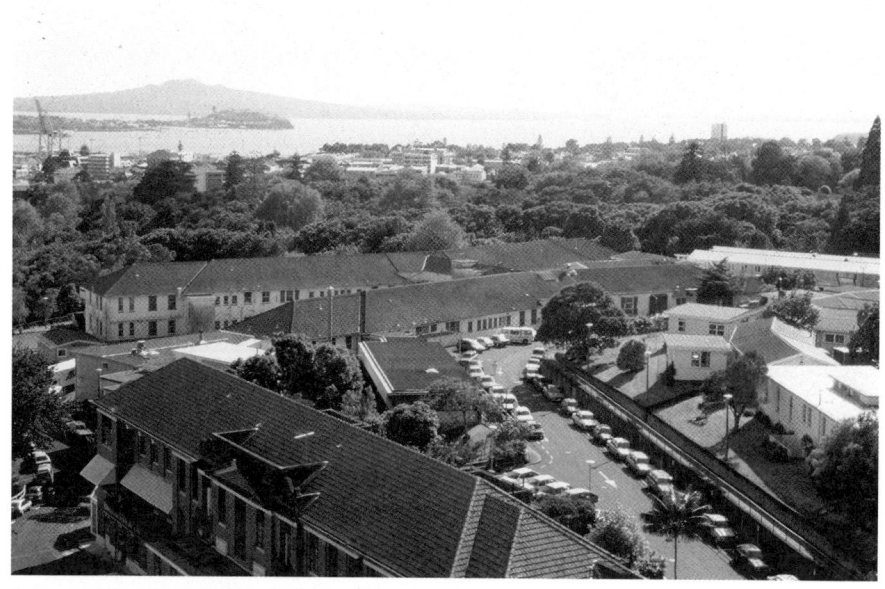

Princess Mary Hospital in the late 1980s, Auckland.
COURTESY OF TE WHĀNAU O IRĀKEWA

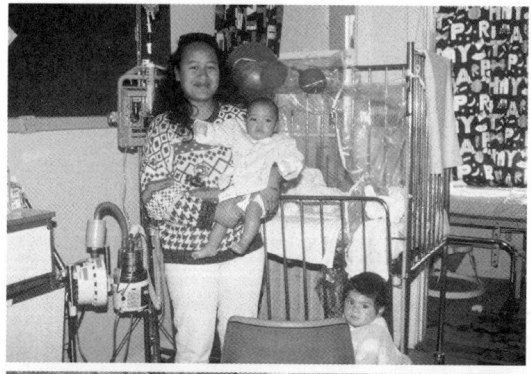

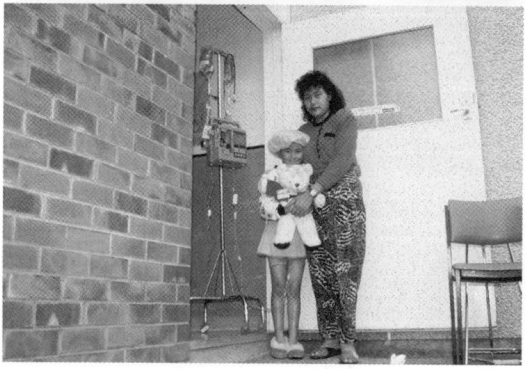

Children and their parents who were guests at Princess Mary Hospital. Sourced from *Te Whanau Atawhai, A New Initiative in Health Provision*, 1993, image collection.
COURTESY OF TE WHĀNAU O IRĀKEWA

APPENDIX 2

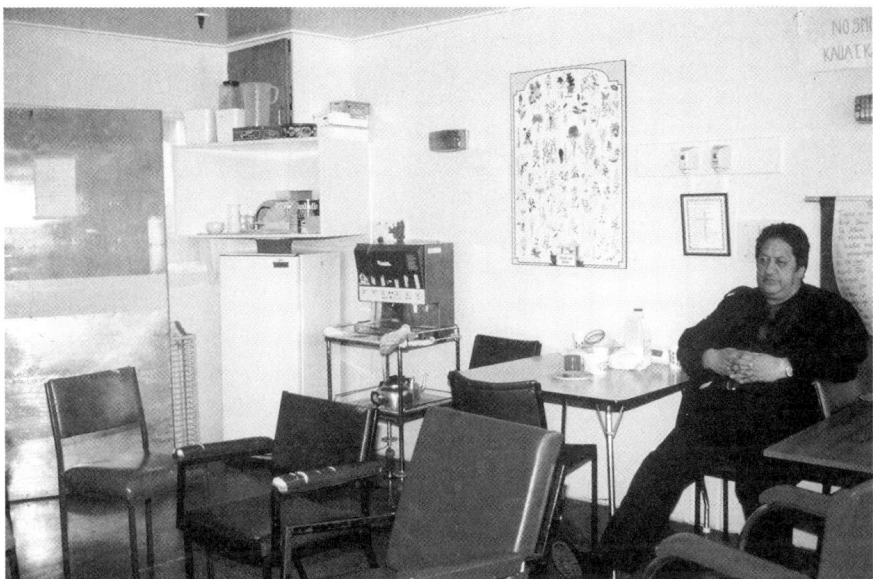

Kaumātua Brownie Williams of Mataatua Marae at Māngere who, along with others, volunteered his services to visit Māori patients and their whānau at Princess Mary Hospital. He saw Whānau Atawhai as a 'mini mobile marae' that ensured the hospital system was sensitive to Māori needs.
COURTESY OF TE WHĀNAU O IRĀKEWA

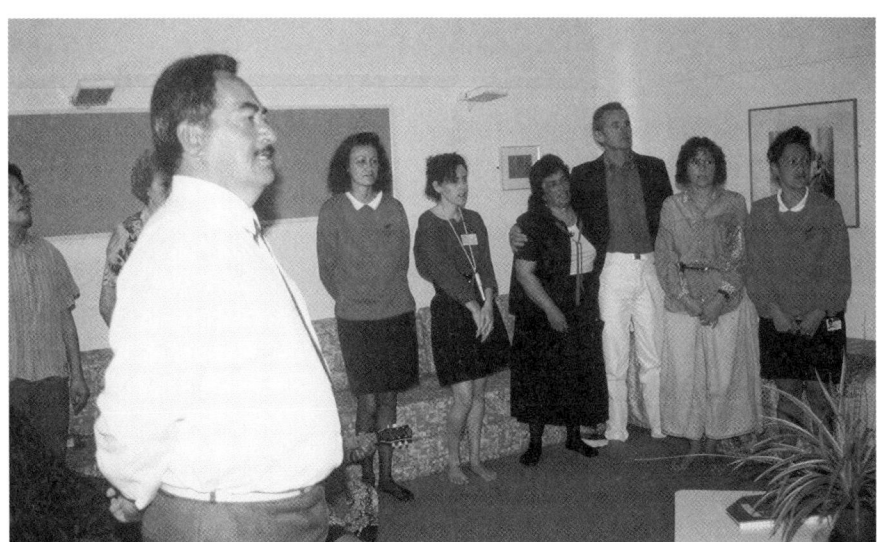

Kaumātua Aronia Ahomiro leads a ceremony with Princess Mary Hospital staff.
COURTESY OF TE WHĀNAU O IRĀKEWA

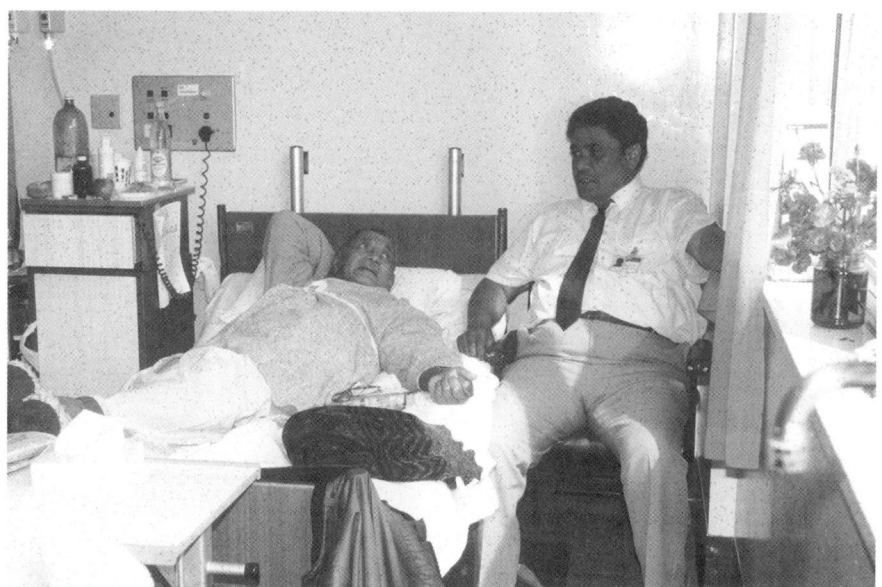

Volunteer kaumātua Rangi Matehaere visiting John Ngamanu, a patient in Auckland Hospital.
COURTESY OF TE WHĀNAU O IRĀKEWA

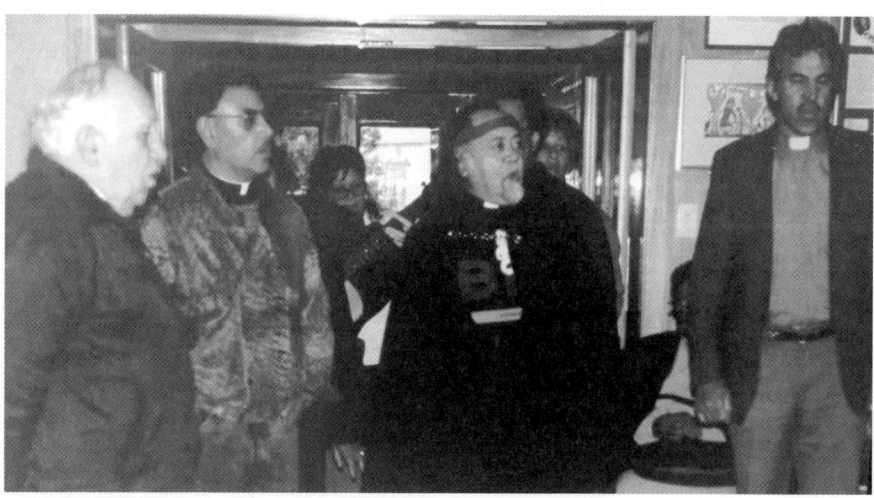

Māori chaplains and tribal representatives were present at the blessing for the opening of Starship Hospital. Pictured here at the reception held in the Marion Davis Centre are Canon John Tamahori, Rev. Wally Te Ua, Rev. Eru Potaka Dewes and Rev. Nehe Dewes.
COURTESY OF TE WHĀNAU O IRĀKEWA

APPENDIX 2

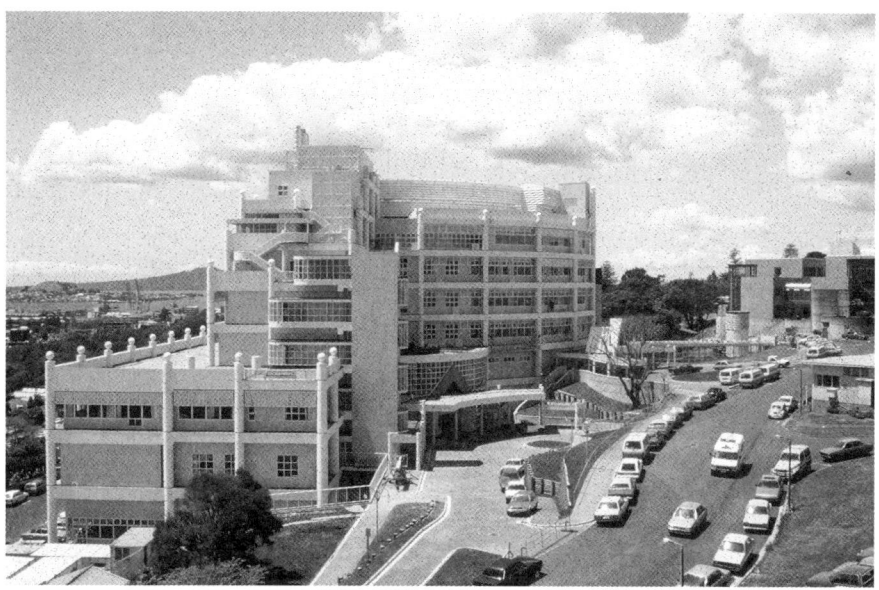

The new Starship Hospital that replaced Princess Mary Hospital. It was opened in 1991 with Māori protocols and officially named in 1992.
COURTESY OF TE WHĀNAU O IRĀKEWA

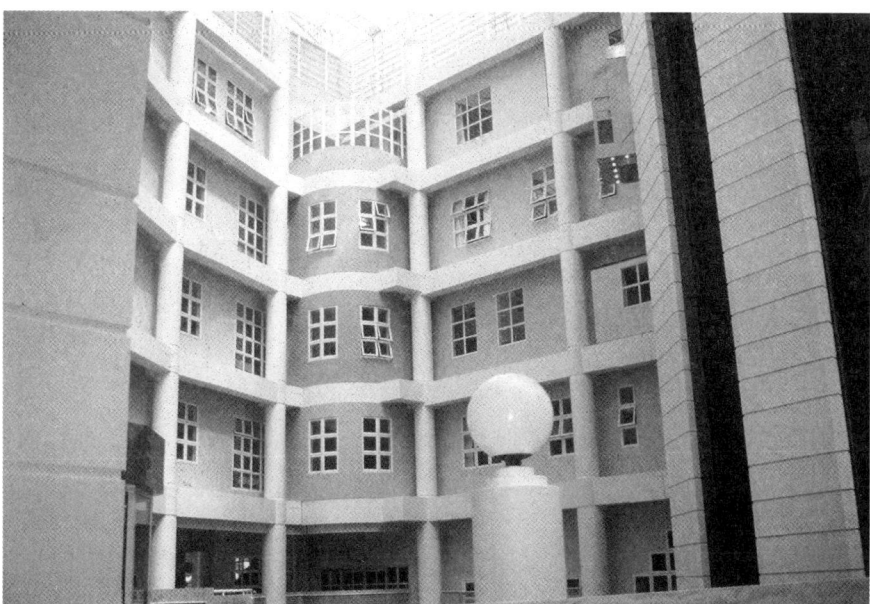

The interior of Starship Hospital.
COURTESY OF TE WHĀNAU O IRĀKEWA

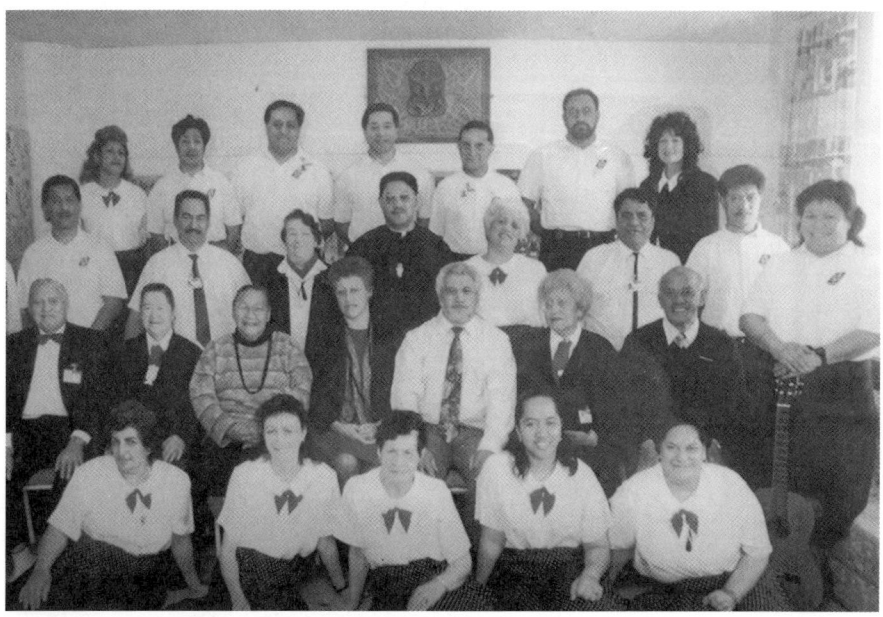

Te Whānau Atawhai team of Starship Hospital, Princess Mary Hospital and Auckland Hospital, 1991.

Back row L-R: Lorvinia George, Whitiao Bristow, Max Bishop, Paora Mathews, Graeme Smith, Lani Mārama, Karena Way.

2nd row L-R: Wiremu Smith, Aronia Ahomiro, Mata Forbes, Rev. Wally Te Ua, Ngapine Brown, Rangi Matehaere, Frank Wiki, Lisa Leger.

3rd Row L-R: Mita Makiha, Monica Rogers, Ruby Gray, Amohaere Ngaropo (Tangitu), Toby Curtis, Lucy Rivers, Bill Tāpuke.

Front Row L-R: Lullita Samuels, Vyna Wiki, Cecelia Burkhart, Rowyne Pai, Renata Hutchinson.

COURTESY OF TE WHĀNAU O IRĀKEWA

APPENDIX 2

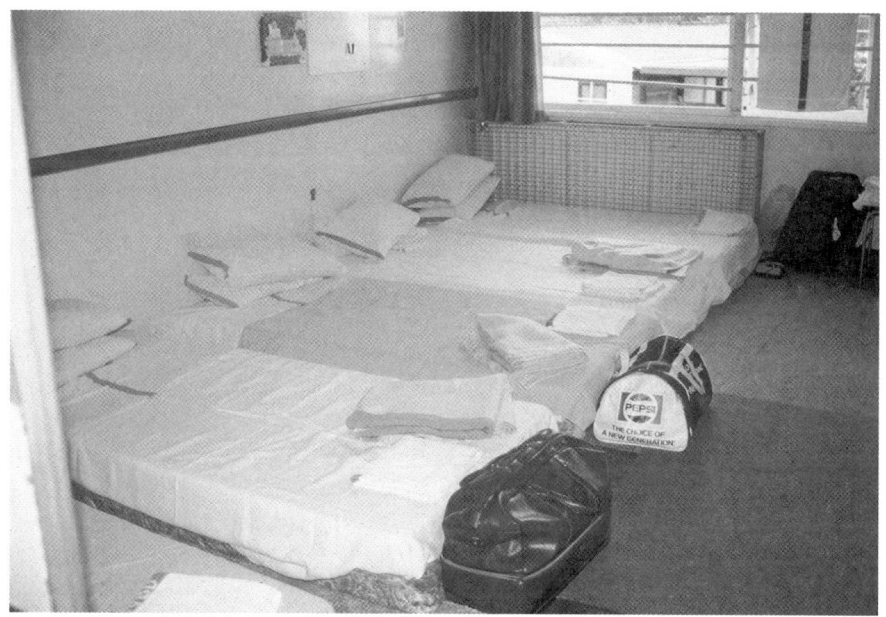

The Whānau Room laid out with matresses marae style in
Te Whānau Atawhai Unit on the seventh floor of Starship Hospital.
COURTESY OF TE WHĀNAU O IRĀKEWA

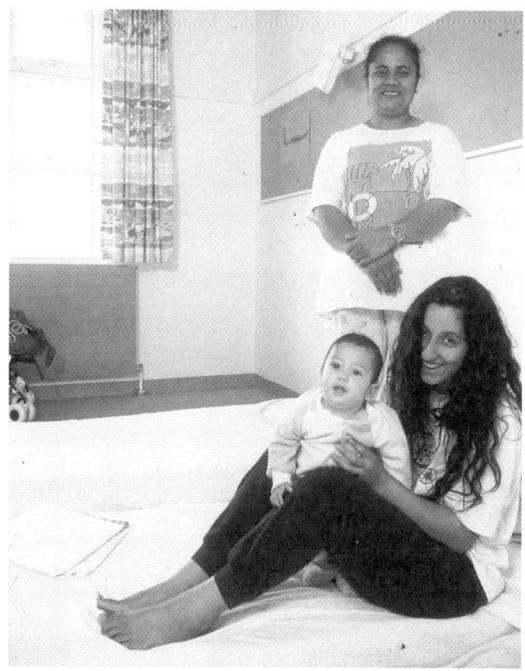

Happy faces at Starship
Hospital with Te Whānau
Atawhai care. Sourced
from *Te Whanau Atawhai,
A New Initiative in Health
Provision*, 1993, image
collection.
COURTESY OF TE WHĀNAU
O IRĀKEWA

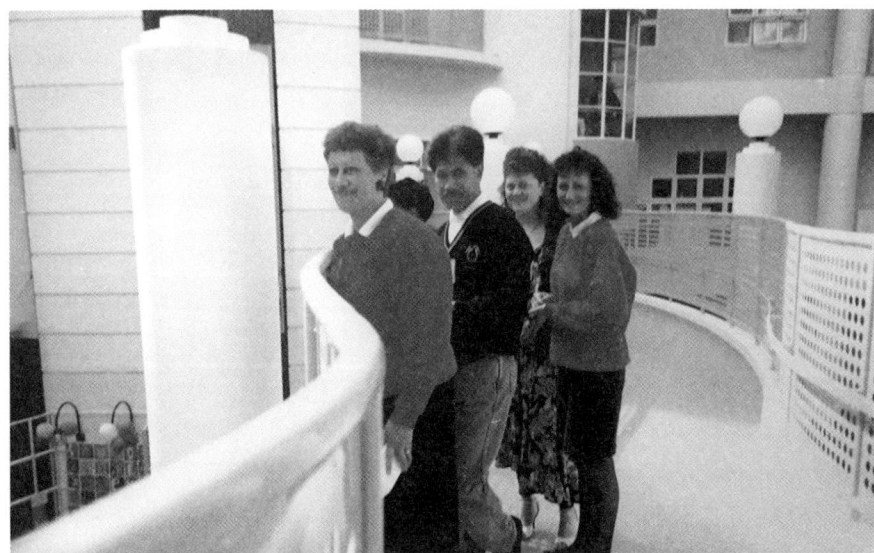

An open day at Starship Hospital with Amohaere Tangitu, Frank Wiki, Vyna Wiki and visitors.
COURTESY OF TE WHĀNAU O IRĀKEWA

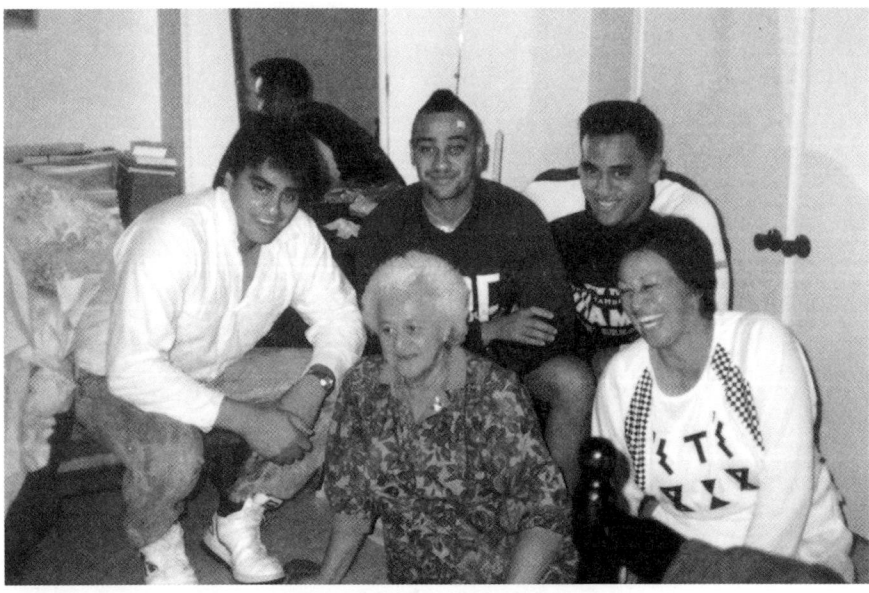

Amohaere with her mother, Mihipeka (Mary) Moanaroa Tangitu (née Gardiner), and her sons (L–R): Samuel, Nicholas (Pouroto) and Christian. (Tamehana absent)
COURTESY OF AMOHAERE TANGITU

APPENDIX 2

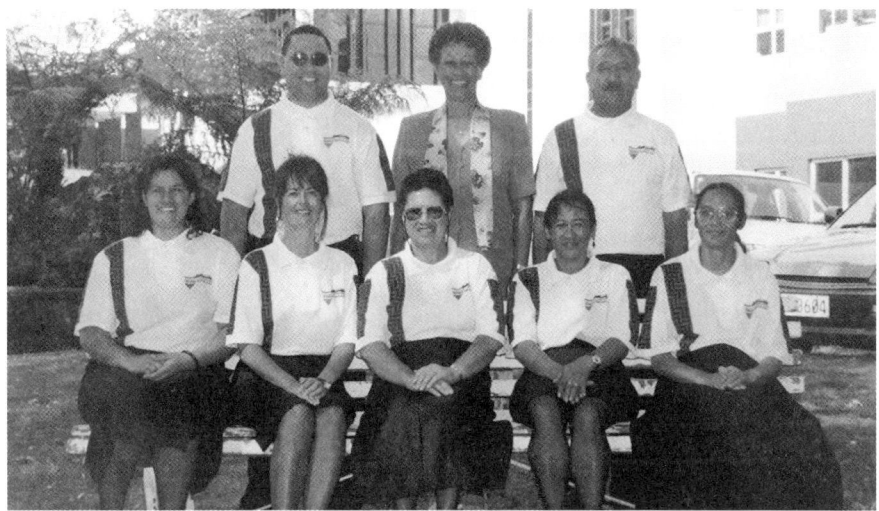

Hunga Manaaki Rotorua team of 1997.
Back row: Michael Naera, Amohaere Ngaropo, Rangitakatū Mihaka.
Front row: Marleina Grant, Cathy Williams, Terewai Heretini, Sue Westbrook, Shona Faulkner.
COURTESY OF TE WHĀNAU O IRĀKEWA

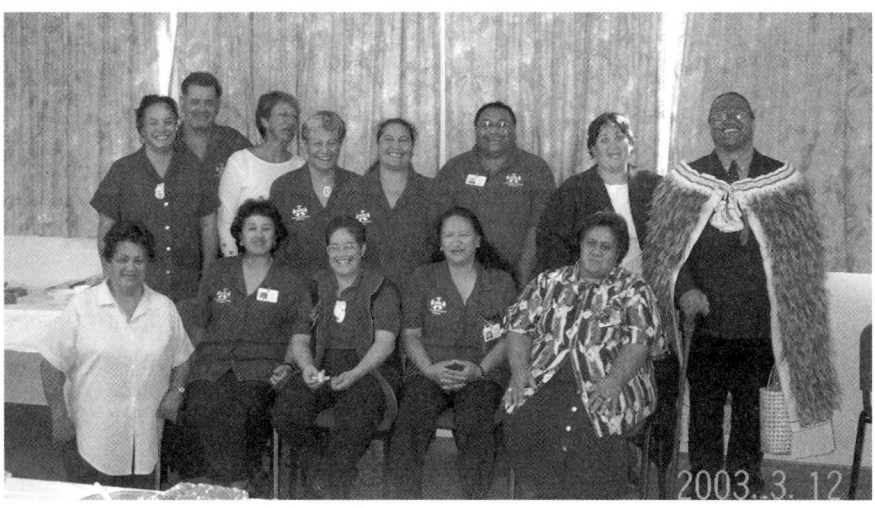

Māori Health Services team 2003 at Pouroto Ngaropo's farewell.
Back row L-R: Titihuia Moses, Tom Chapman, Amohaere Tangitu, Tupari Clay, Kahuariki Hancock, Arameina Heihei, Mary Rio, Pouroto Ngaropo.
Front row L-R: Ronnie Kouka, Riripeti Rio, Heeni Taukamo, Mereana White, Terehia Kira.
COURTESY OF TE WHĀNAU O IRĀKEWA

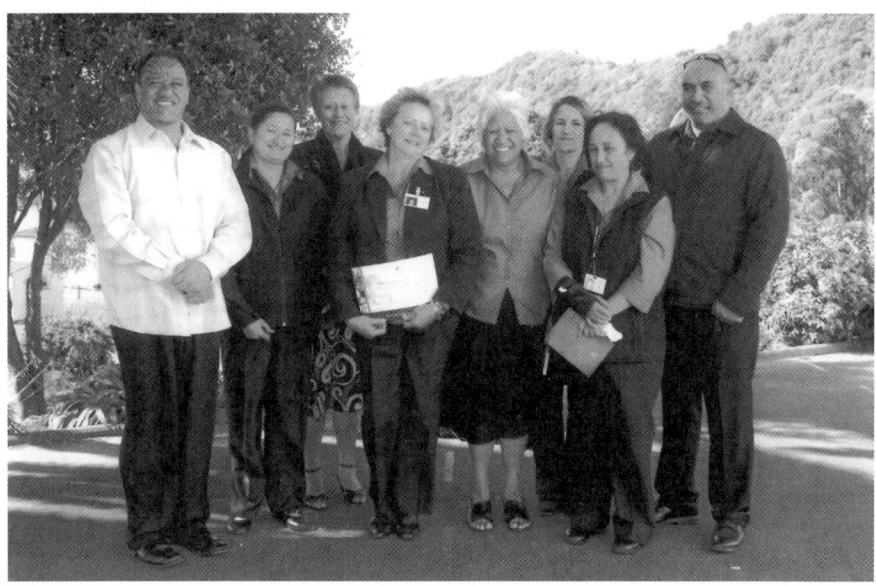

Staff recognition for Te Whānau o Irākewa, 2009. L–R: Pouroto Ngaropo, Hīria Hōhua, Amohaere Tangitu, Astrid Tawhai (recipient), Ngamihi Crapp, Hineatakura Strum, Riripeti Rio, Lani Mārama.
COURTESY OF TE WHĀNAU O IRAKEWA

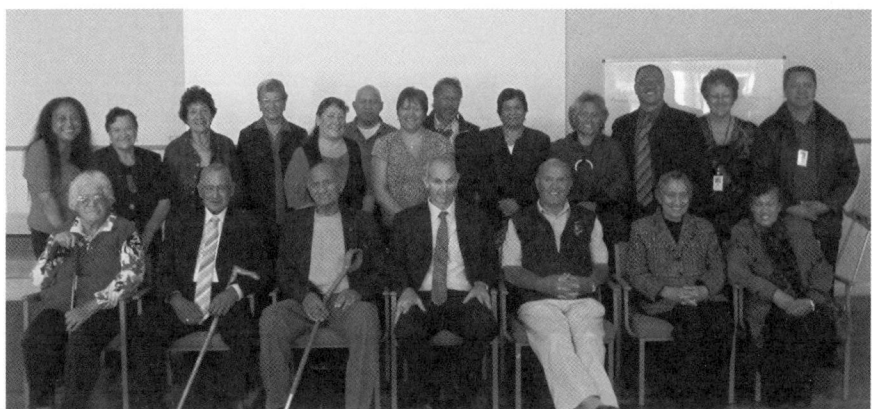

The 2012 Kāhui Kaumātua council representing eighteen tribes was formed when the Eastbay Health and Western Bay of Plenty Health districts merged.
COURTESY OF TE WHĀNAU O IRĀKEWA

APPENDIX 2

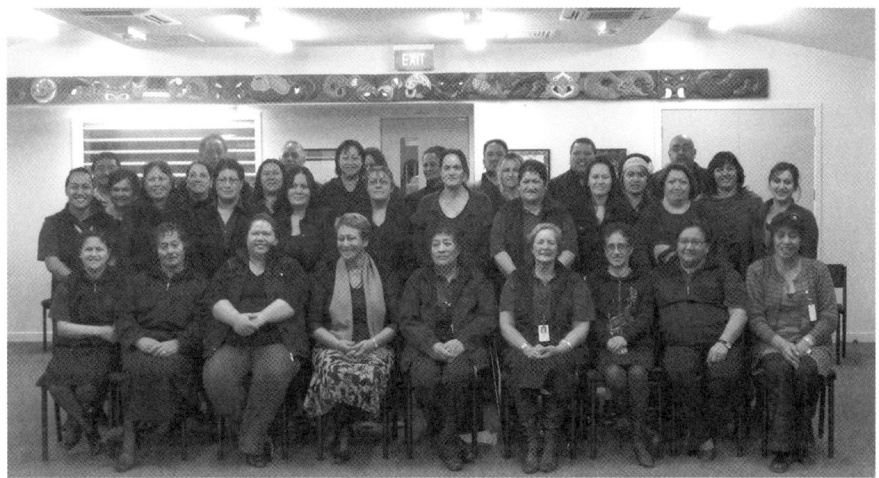

Amohaere and the full Te Whānau o Irākewa Māori Health Services team for 2010.
COURTESY OF TE WHĀNAU O IRĀKEWA

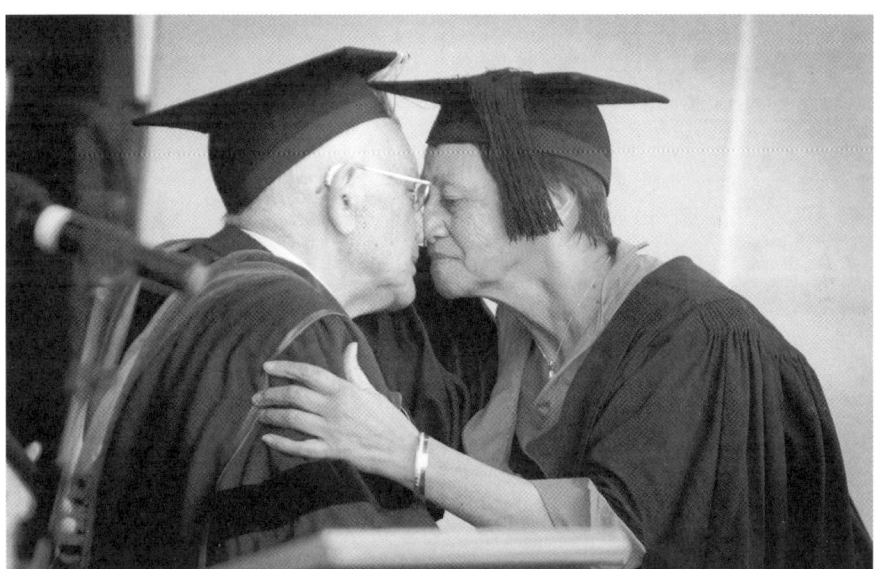

Amohaere receives an award in December 2012 as a Distinguished Fellow – Māori Health Sciences (Nursing) from Te Whare Wānanga o Awanuiārangi Chairperson Distinguished Professor Sir Sidney Mead (Hirini Moko Mead).
COURTESY OF TE WHARE WĀNANGA O AWANUIĀRANGI

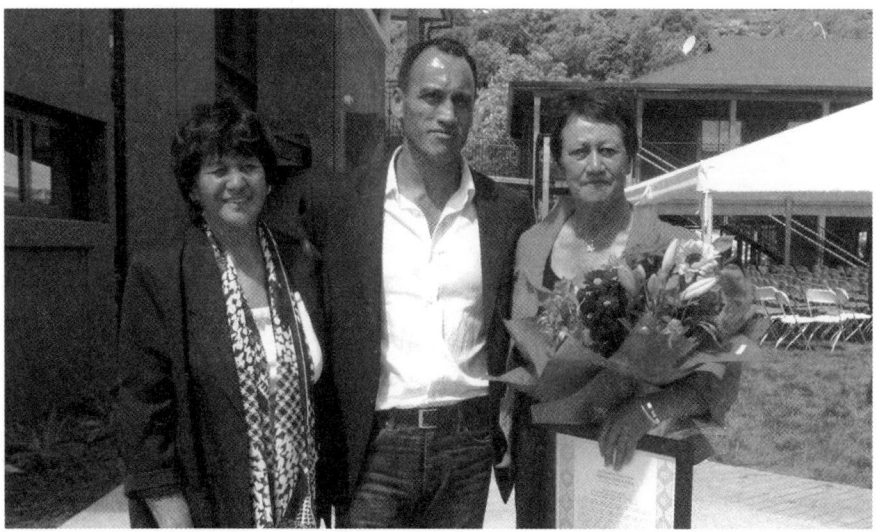

Amohaere with her son Christian and Gwen Tuhimate at the 2012 ceremony where she received the distinguished fellow award in 2012.
COURTESY OF TE WHĀNAU O IRĀKEWA

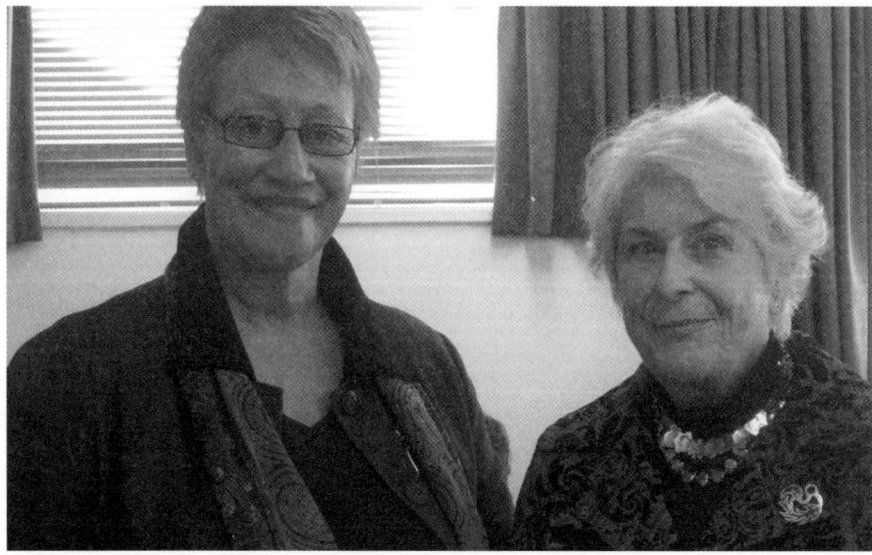

Amohaere with Mary Hackett CNZM, Chairperson for the Bay of Plenty District Health Board (2001-2010). In her earlier role as Principal Nurse at Auckland Hospital, Mary Hackett, then known as Nurse Futter, opened the door for biculturalism and cultural safety to enter Auckland Hospital, which led to Amohaere's first hospital position as the Bicultural Parent Liaison Officer in 1987.
COURTESY OF TE WHĀNAU O IRĀKEWA

ENDNOTES

Intro

1. Mason Durie, *Mauri Ora: The Dynamics of Māori Health* (Auckland, NZ: Oxford University Press, 2001), 49.
2. Mason Durie, *Whaiora: Māori Health Development*. 2nd ed. (Auckland, NZ: Oxford University Press, 1998), 61.
3. Mason Durie, 'Māori Health Transitions 1960–1985,' in *Huia Histories of Māori Ngā Tāhuhu Kōrero*, ed. Danny Keenan (Wellington, NZ: Huia Publishers, 2012), 267.
4. Mere Roberts, 'Revisiting "The Natural World of the Māori",' in *Huia Histories of Māori: Ngā Tāhuhu Kōrero*, ed. Danny Keenan (Wellington, NZ: Huia Publishers, 2012), 53.
5. Ibid.
6. Elaine Papps and Irihapeti Ramsden, 'Cultural Safety in Nursing: The New Zealand Experience,' *International Journal for Quality in Health Care*, no. 5 (1996): 496.
7. 'Judith Amohaere Tangitu Distinguished Fellow – Māori Health Sciences (Nursing),' *Pū Kāea*, October–November 2012, 13. http://tumekefm.co.nz/wp-content/uploads/2012/12/Pu-Kaea-Oct-Nov-2012-com.pdf (accessed 9 July 2018).

Chapter 1

1. Henare Arekatera Tate, 'Towards Some Foundations of a Systematic Māori Theology He Tirohanga Anganui Ki Ētahi Kaupapa Hōhonu Mō Te Whakapono Māori' (Doctorate of Philosophy, Melbourne College of Divinity, 2010), section 6.3.1.2.1, 175–178.
2. Mason Durie, *Whaiora: Māori Health Development.*, 2nd ed. (Auckland, NZ: Oxford University Press, 1998), 70.

Chapter 2

1. 'Mrs Te Amohaere Gardiner,' *Te Ao Hou The New World*, no. 42 (March 1963), http://teaohou.natlib.govt.nz/journals/teaohou/issue/Mao42TeA/c34.html (accessed 10 November 2014).
2. Alexandra McKegg, 'Cameron, Robina Thomson,' *The Dictionary of New Zealand Biography*. *Te Ara – the Encyclopedia of New Zealand*, Wellington, NZ: Ministry of Culture and Heritage, June 6, 2013, http://www.teara.govt.nz/en/biographies/4c2/cameron-robina-thomson (accessed 6 June 2013).
3. Mason Durie, *Whaiora: Māori Health Development*. 2nd ed. (Auckland, NZ: Oxford University Press 1998), 47.
4. *Te Ao Hou The New World*, no. 42 (March 1963), http://teaohou.natlib.govt.nz/journals/teaohou/issue/Mao42TeA/c34.html (accessed 10 November 2014).
5. Personal comment to author by Sir Wira Gardiner, Whakatāne, 13 December 2014.
6. Personal comment to author by Toby Curtis, Rotorua, 25 March 2015.

7. R. Barker, 'Kia Koutou' (1988), quoted in *Māori Mental Health: Past Trends, Current Issues, and Māori Responsiveness*, Te Kani Kingi (Wellington, NZ: Te Pūmanawa Hauora, Research School of Public Health, Massey University, 2005), 10.

Chapter 3

1. Paul Meredith, 'Urban Maori as "New Citizens": The Quest for Recognition and Resources,' in *Re Visioning Citizenship for the 21st Century, Proceedings of Re Visioning Citizenship for the 21st Century Conference*, eds P. Havemann and G. Morgan (Hamilton: School of Law, University of Waikato, 2000), 3.
2. Melissa Matutina Williams, *Pangaru and the City: Kāinga Tahi, Kāinga Rua. An Urban Migration History* (Wellington, NZ: Bridget Williams Books, 2015), 172.
3. Kerryn Pollock. 'Children's homes and fostering – Government institutions,' *Te Ara – the Encyclopedia of New Zealand*, 5 May 2011, http://www.TeAra.govt.nz/en/childrens-homes-and-fostering/page-2 (accessed 12 July 2018).
4. *Puao-Te-Ata-Tu (Day Break) The Report of the Ministerial Advisory Committee on a Māori Perspective for the Department of Social Welfare* (Wellington, NZ: Department of Social Welfare, June 1986), 2.
5. Ibid, 7.
6. Ibid, 16.
7. Ibid, 7.
8. Ibid, 15.

Chapter 4

1. Stephenie Knight, *Auckland Hospital Racism Intervention Project, A History* (Auckland, NZ: Race Relations Office and Auckland Hospital Board, 1989), 8.
2. Ibid, 5.
3. Personal comment to author by Karena Way, Auckland, 22 August 2017.
4. Stephenie Knight, 1989, op. cit., 5, 12.
5. Ibid, 5.
6. Ibid, 6.
7. Personal comment to author by Karena Way, Auckland, 4 October 2017. See also Stephenie Knight, 1989, op. cit., 12.
8. Stephenie Knight, 1989, op. cit., 7.
9. Ibid, 15–17.
10. *Puao-Te-Ata-Tu (Day Break) The Report of the Ministerial Advisory Committee on a Māori Perspective for the Department of Social Welfare* (Wellington, NZ: Department of Social Welfare, June 1986), 18.
11. Stephenie Knight, 1989, op. cit., 3.
12. Margaret Mutu, *The State of Māori Rights* (Wellington, NZ: Huia Publishers, 2011), 3.
13. *A Fair Go for All? Rite Tahi Tatou Katoa? Addressing Structural Discrimination in Public Services, A Discussion Paper by the Human Rights Commission* (Wellington, NZ: Human Rights Commission, July 2012), 3, https://www.hrc.co.nz/files/2914/2409/4608/HRC-Structural-Report_final_webV1.pdf (accessed 9 July 2018).
14. Amohaere G. Ngaropo, B. J. Anderson, and K. Way, 'Te Whānau Atawhai: A New Zealand Model For Supporting Indigenous Families With Children in Intensive Care' (presentation, 1990), 3.
15. *A Fair Go for All? Rite Tahi Tatou Katoa? Addressing Structural Discrimination in Public Services, A Discussion Paper by the Human Rights Commission*, 2012, op. cit., 4.
16. See State Owned Enterprises Act, 1986, section 9 The Treaty.

17. Mason Durie, 'The Treaty of Waitangi and Health Care,' *New Zealand Medical Journal*, no. 102 (1989): 293.
18. Ibid.
19. Ibid.
20. Ibid. See also Lyndon Keene, 'Working Against Racism,' *New Zealand Nursing Journal*, 81 (August 1988): 18.
21. Mason Durie, 1989, op. cit., 284.
22. Nurse Mary Futter was later known as Mary Hackett.
23. Heather Thompson, Auckland Area Health Board, phone interview with author, 22 June 2015. Heather mentioned Principal Nurse Mary Hackett as a key advocate in bringing a more Māori culturally sensitive understanding to hospital treatment.
24. Personal comment to author by Karena Way, Auckland, 4 October 2017.
25. Personal comment to author by Ron Dunham, Rotorua, 24 March 2015.
26. Personal comment to author by Toby Curtis, Rotorua, 25 March 2015.
27. 'Whānau Accommodation – Te Whare Awhina,' Starship Hospital, 2015, https://www.starship.org.nz/patients-parents-and-visitors/whats-at-starship/places-to-stay/whanau-accommodation-te-whare-awhina/ (accessed 10 October 2018).

Chapter 5

1. Pipi Barton, '"A Kind of Ritual Pākehā Tikanga" – Māori Experiences of Hospitalisation: A Case Study,' (Master of Philosophy in Nursing, Massey University, Albany, New Zealand, 2008), 31.
2. Ibid.
3. Derek A. Dow, *Māori Health and Government Policy 1840–1940* (Wellington, NZ: Victoria University Press, 1999), 74.
4. Ibid.
5. Golan Maaka, 'Health Trends in Māori Today,' a paper for the Young Māori Leaders Conference in 1959, in *Dr Golan Maaka Māori Doctor*, Bradford Haami (Auckland, NZ: Tandem Press, 1995), 147.
6. Ibid.
7. Ibid.
8. Henare Arekatera Tate, 'Towards Some Foundations of a Systematic Māori Theology He Tirohanga Anganui Ki Ētahi Kaupapa Hōhonu Mō Te Whakapono Māori' (Doctorate of Philosophy, Melbourne College of Divinity, 2010), section 6.3.1.2.1, 175–178.
9. The docks of a number of hospitals had to be rennovated for the same reason.
10. Personal comment to author by Ron Dunham (past General Manager Auckland Hospital), Rotorua, 24 March 2015.
11. Patrick Michael Whittle, 'Darwinism and the Nature of Māori,' *MAI Review*, (2009): 5.
12. Elaine Papps and Irihapeti Ramsden, 'Cultural Safety in Nursing: The New Zealand Experience,' *International Journal for Quality in Health Care*, no. 5 (1996): 493.
13. *Guidelines for Cultural Safety, the Treaty of Waitangi and Mari Health in Nursing Education and Practice* (Wellington, NZ: Nursing Council of New Zealand, 2011), 6, http://pro.healthmentoronline.com/assets/Uploads/refract/pdf/Nursing_Council_cultural-safety11.pdf (accessed 9 July 2018).
14. Stephenie Knight, *Auckland Hospital Racism Intervention Project, A History* (Auckland, NZ: Race Relations Office and Auckland Hospital Board, 1989), 8.
15. Amohaere Gardiner Tangitu, '*Annual Report of the Māori Liaison Officer*' (Auckland, NZ: Princess Mary Hospital, 5 July 1989).
16. Stephenie Knight, op. cit., 19.

17. Ibid, 9.
18. Personal comment to author by Dr John Newman, Auckland, 2016.
19. Stephenie Knight, 1989, op. cit., 16.
20. Ibid.
21. Ibid, 9.
22. Amohaere Gardiner Tangitū, 1989, op. cit.

Chapter 6

1. Canon John Tamahori, 'Māori Education,' *Te Ao Hou The New World*, (1 January 1972): 24.
2. *Auckland Sales and Hospital Endowments, Waitangi Tribunal Report 261* (Wellington, NZ: Waitangi Tribunal, Department of Justice, 1991), 2–3, https://forms.justice.govt.nz/search/Documents/WT/wt_DOC_68359805/Interim%20Report%20on%20Auckland%20Hospital%20Endowments.pdf (accessed 9 July 2018).
3. Ibid.
4. Ibid.
5. Rina Moore, 'The State of Māori Health,' *Te Ao Hou The New World*, (1960): 8.
6. See further discussion on this in; Henare Arekatera Tate, *He Puna Iti I Te Ao Mārama A Little Spring in the World of Light* (Auckland, NZ: Libro International, 2012).
7. Mason Durie, *Whaiora: Māori Health Development*. 2nd ed. (Auckland, NZ: Oxford University Press, 1998), 134.
8. Ibid.

Chapter 7

1. *The Oxford English Dictionary* (UK: Oxford University Press, 2002).
2. John C. Moorfield, *Māori Dictionary, Te Aka English–Māori, Māori–English Dictionary and Index* (New Zealand, 2016, 2003), māoridictionary.co.nz.
3. *Best Health Outcomes for Māori: Practice Implications* (Wellington, NZ: Medical Council of New Zealand, 2008), 2.
4. Ibid, 24.
5. Amohaere G. Ngaropo, B. J. Anderson, and K. Way, 'Te Whānau Atawhai: A New Zealand Model For Supporting Indigenous Families With Children in Intensive Care' (presentation, 1990), 5.
6. *Best Health Outcomes for Māori: Practice Implications*, 2008, op. cit., 29.

Chapter 8

1. Mason Durie, *Whaiora: Māori Health Development*. 2nd ed. (Auckland, NZ: Oxford University Press, 1998), 69.
2. Mason Durie, 'Pae Ora: Māori Health Horizons', Massey University Te Mata o Te Tau Lecture Series 2009, 7 July 2009, 3. http://www.manu-ao.ac.nz/massey/fms/manu-ao/documents/Pae%20Ora%20-%20Maori%20Health%20Horizons.pdf?B76AC0F2A1EF64CD377ADD13B162624E (accessed 9 July 2018).
3. Mason Durie, 1998, op. cit., 72–76.
4. Mason Durie, 2009, op. cit., 4
5. Mason Durie, 1998, op. cit., 76.
6. *Report of the Committee of Inquiry into the Death at Carrington Hospital of Manihera Mansel Watene and Other Related Matters* (Wellington, NZ: Department of Health, July 1991), 19, http://www.moh.govt.nz/notebook/nbbooks.nsf/0/6D27C1C11347822F4C2565D7000DEE34/$file/Report_Committee_Inquiry_death_Carrington_Hospital.pdf (accessed 9 July 2018); Mason Durie in Te Kani Kingi et al, *Maea Te Toi Ora: Māori Health Transformations* (Wellington, NZ: Huia Publishers, 2018).

7. Mason Durie, 1998, op. cit., 153–154
8. Mason Durie, 2009, op. cit., 3.
9. *Guidelines for Cultural Safety, the Treaty of Waitangi and Māori Health in Nursing Education and Practice* (Wellington, NZ: Nursing Council of New Zealand, 2011), 6, http://pro.healthmentoronline.com/assets/Uploads/refract/pdf/Nursing_Council_cultural-safety11.pdf (accessed 9 July 2018).
10. Elaine Papps and Irihapeti Ramsden, 'Cultural Safety in Nursing: The New Zealand Experience,' *International Journal for Quality in Health Care*, no. 5 (1996): 491.
11. Ibid, 495.
12. Ibid, 496.
13. Ibid, 493.
14. Mason Durie, 1998, op. cit., 114.
15. Ibid, 77.
16. Ibid, 78.
17. *Te Whānau Atawhai, A New Initiative in Health Provision* (Auckland, NZ: Te Whānau Atawhai, 1993), 5.
18. Ibid.
19. Personal comment to author by Dr John Newman, Auckland, 2016.
20. Rina Moore, 'The State of Māori Health,' *Te Ao Hou The New World*, no. 33, (1960): 6–11.
21. Ibid.
22. Personal comment to author by Dr John Newmann, Auckland, 2016.
23. Rina Moore, 1960, op. cit., 2.
24. 'Starship Hospital Celebrates 21st Anniversary,' *New Zealand Herald*, 16 November 2012.
25. R.A. Kearns and J.R. Barnett, 'Happy Meals in the Starship Enterprise; Interpreting a Moral Geography of Health Care Consumption,' *Health and Place 6*, no. 2 (2000): 85.
26. 'Steps into the Future. Te Whānau Atawhai Developments to the Year 2000' (Te Whānau Atawhai Archive, February 1992), 9.
27. Ibid.

Chapter 9

1. Peter Calder, 'A Rough Road to Unity,' *New Zealand Herald*, 15 December 1990.
2. Ibid.
3. 'Steps into the Future. Te Whānau Atawhai Developments to the Year 2000' (Te Whānau Atawhai Archive, February 1992), 12.
4. *Te Whānau Atawhai Annual Report – 1992* (Auckland, NZ: Starship Hospital, October 1992), 8.
5. Ibid.
6. Ibid, 7.
7. Ibid, 8.
8. Ibid.
9. Ibid.
10. Ibid, 7.
11. Ibid. See also 'Te Whānau Atawhai Meeting Minutes 9 September 1992' (Auckland, NZ: Te Whānau Atawhai Archive, Starship Hospital, 9 September 1992), 3.
12. 'Te Whānau Atawhai Meeting Minutes 9 September 1992,' op. cit.
13. *Te Whānau Atawhai Annual Report – 1992*, op. cit., 7.
14. Auckland Area Health Board Job Description, 5 July 1989.
15. *Te Whānau Atawhai Annual Report – 1992*, op. cit., 4.

16. Ibid.
17. Ibid, 2, 7–8.
18. Mason Durie, *Maori Cultural Competencies for Health and Disability Advocates* (Wellington, NZ: Health and Disability Advocacy, Nga Kaitautoko, 2006), 2, http://advocacy.hdc.org.nz/media/146523/m%C3%A4ori%20cultural%20competencies%20for%20health%20and%20disability%20advocates.pdf (accessed 10 October 2018).
19. *Te Whānau Atawhai Annual Report – 1992*, op, cit.
20. 'Steps into the Future. Te Whānau Atawhai Developments to the Year 2000,' 1992, op. cit., 1–5.
21. 'Te Whānau Atawhai Meeting Minutes 9 September 1992,' op. cit., 3.
22. *Te Whānau Atawhai Annual Report – 1992*, op. cit., 10.
23. Ibid, 11.
24. 'Te Whānau Atawhai Meeting Minutes 9 September 1992,' op. cit., 4.
25. *Te Whānau Atawhai, A New Initiative in Health Provision* (Auckland, NZ: Te Whānau Atawhai, 1993), 8–9.
26. Amohaere G. Ngaropo, B. J. Anderson, and K. Way, 'Te Whānau Atawhai: A New Zealand Model For Supporting Indigenous Families With Children in Intensive Care' (presentation, 1990), 8.
27. *Cartwright Inquiry, The Facts about the Cartwright Inquiry*, 7 December 2011, http://www.cartwrightinquiry.com/ (accessed 23 March 2016).
28. Ibid.
29. 'The Cartwright Report,' *Cartwright Inquiry, The Facts about the Cartwright Inquiry*, 5 August 1988, http://www.cartwrightinquiry.com/?page_id=105 (accessed 23 March 2016), 159, 160, 171, 173, 180.
30. Amohaere G. Ngaropo, 'Te Whānau Atawhai Integration of Te Whānau Atawhai with Greenlane and National Womens Hospitals, A Proposal to North Health,' (Auckland, NZ: Te Whānau Atawhai Archive, July 1994).
31. *Te Whānau Atawhai, A New Initiative in Health Provision* (Auckland, NZ: Te Whānau Atawhai, 1993), 12–13.
32. Toby Curtis, 'Letter to Dennis Pickup Chief Executive for Auckland Healthcare' (Te Whānau Atawhai Archive, Starship Hospital, 18 March 1994).
33. 'Te Whānau Atawhai Committee Meeting 16 March 1994' (Auckland, NZ: Te Whānau Atawhai Archive, Starship Hospital, 16 March 1994), 3–4.
34. Amohaere Tangitu Ngaropo and Naida Pou, 'He Kamaka Oranga Strategic Plan 1993/1994, Māori Health Management Developments to the Year 2000' (He Kamaka Oranga, 1994), 4.
35. Ibid, 3.
36. Ibid.
37. Ibid, 4.
38. Ibid, 4, 7.
39. Ibid, slide 15.
40. Ibid, slide 17.
41. 'Te Whānau Atawhai Committee Meeting 16 March 1994,' op. cit., 4.
42. 'Auckland Hospital Publication of Nursing Policy and Standards of Practice' (Auckland Healthcare, March 1994), 18–19.
43. Ibid.
44. Ibid.
45. 'Hospital Pioneer Says Farewell,' *Nga Korero o Te Wa*, August 1994.
46. 'He Kamaka Oranga Maori Health at ADHB,' *Nova Te Whetumarama, Te Pānui Mō Ngā Kaimahi a Te Toka Tumai* (July 2006): 5.

Chapter 10

1. 'Māori Health Development' (Rotorua, NZ: Lakes District Health Board, 13 June 2013), http://www.lakesdhb.govt.nz/Article.aspx?ID=2599.
2. Ibid.
3. Ibid.
4. 'Hunga Manaaki – Celebrating 10 Years of Service at Rotorua Hospital' (Rotorua, NZ: Lakes District Health Board and Hunga Manaaki, March 2007), 1, http://www.lakesdhb.govt.nz/Resource.aspx?ID=7286
5. Ibid, 6.
6. Ibid, 5.
7. Ibid.
8. Ibid.
9. 'Healthy Communities Mauriora' (Lakes District Health Board, 13 June 2013), http://www.lakesdhb.govt.nz/Article.aspx?ID=2599 (accessed 24 June 2017).
10. 'Haven of Peace,' *Rotorua Review*, 31 January 1995.
11. 'Hunga Manaaki – Celebrating 10 Years of Service at Rotorua Hospital', 2007, op. cit., 1.
12. Ibid.
13. Ibid, 7.
14. Ibid, 1.
15. Ibid, 7.
16. Ibid, 3.
17. Ibid, 4.
18. Ibid.
19. Ibid.
20. Ibid.
21. Ibid.
22. Ibid, 7.
23. Ibid.
24. Ibid.
25. Ibid.
26. Ibid.
27. Ibid.
28. Stephanie Arthur-Worsop, 'Tears at Decision to End Maori Support Service at Hospital,' *New Zealand Herald*, 9 June 2017, http://www.nzherald.co.nz/nz/news/article.cfm?c_id=1&objectid=11873173. (accessed 11 June 2017).
29. Hauora o Te Moana Nui a Toi Bay of Plenty District Māori Health Services Iwi Consultation Report 2010, 6.

Chapter 11

1. 'Hauora O Te Moana Nui a Toi Bay of Plenty District Health Services Iwi Consultation Report' (Tauranga, NZ: Bay of Plenty District Health Board, 2010), 6.
2. Ibid, 7.
3. Anna Fifield, 'Amohaere Comes Home to Eastern Bay,' *Eastbay News*, 23 April 1998.
4. Ibid.
5. 'Basic Cultural Safety Aspects Stage Three' (Māori Health Services, Whakatāne Hospital, Pacific Health Ltd, 2004), 26.

6. Shirley Whitwell, 'Choice in Māori Health Service,' *Eastbay News*, 28 November 2002.
7. Anna Fifield, 1998, op. cit.
8. 'Hospital Staff Lack "Bicultural Understanding",' *The Whakatāne Beacon*, 29 September 1998. See also Dianne Kopae, 'Health Initiatives Culturally-Friendly,' *Eastbay News*, 4 February 1999.
9. 'Te Tokotoko Poutiriao Te Whānau o Irākewa Staff Orientation Manual,' (Bay of Plenty District Health Board, Whakatāne, 2008), 10.
10. Dianne Kopae, 1999, op. cit.
11. Ibid.
12. *Te Hauora O Te Moana Nui a Toi Pacific Health, Iwi Consultation* (Whakatāne, NZ: Te Whatumauri Hauora Whakatāne Hospital, 2005), 15–16.
13. 'Bay of Plenty District Health Board Hauora A Toi – Your DHB', *Bay of Plenty District Health Board Hauora a Toi*, 14 August 2015, http://www.bopdhb.govt.nz/your-dhb/tauranga-hospital-centenary/m%C4%81ori-health/. See also *Celebrating 100 Years of Innovation and Excellence: Tauranga Hospital 6 March 1914–2014* (Tauranga, NZ: Bay of Plenty District Health Board, 2014), 22, http://tauranga.kete.net.nz/documents/0000/0000/0448/Celebrating_100_years.pdf (accessed 9 July 2018).
14. Tangata Whenua Cultural Safety – Whakatāne, Policy no. 1.4.1, July 2000, in 'Nga Tikanga Whakahaere-a-Tangata Mo Toi Te Ora Cultural Safety. Aspects for Toi Te Ora When Engaging Tangata Whenua Mauriora. Māori Perspectives Relating to Cultural Safety,' Pouroto Ngaropo (Toi te Ora Community Health and Disability Services, Pacific Health, 2003), 1–3. At this time, the New Zealand Health and Disability Act 2000, also acknowledged the special relationship between Māori and the Crown under the Treaty of Waitangi.
15. Blessing Of The Room After A Patient Has Died, Policy no. 1.6.2, April 2001, 'Nga Tikanga Whakahaere-a-Tangata Mo Toi Te Ora Cultural Safety. Aspects for Toi Te Ora When Engaging Tangata Whenua Mauriora. Māori Perspectives Relating to Cultural Safety,' Pouroto Ngaropo (Toi te Ora Community Health and Disability Services, Pacific Health, 2003), 1–3.
16. Ibid, 1.
17. Ibid, 1–3.
18. Shirley Whitwell, 'Choice in Māori Health Service,' op. cit., 2002.
19. Ibid.
20. Pouroto Ngaropo, 'Ngā Poumana O Io Māori Health Services Integration into Toi Te Ora' (Māori Health Services Pacific Health, 11 July 2003), 2.
21. Ibid, 1.
22. Ibid, 3.
23. In 1840, the year the Treaty of Waitangi was signed, Māori were guardians over 66.4 million acres; by 1850 that had halved; by 1890 it was 11 million acres and in 2013 a mere 3.6 million acres.
24. Pouroto Ngaropo, 'Nga Tikanga Whakahaere-a-Tangata Mo Toi Te Ora Cultural Safety. Aspects for Toi Te Ora When Engaging Tangata Whenua Mauriora. Māori Perspectives Relating to Cultural Safety' (Toi te Ora Community Health and Disability Services, Pacific Health, 2003), 10.
25. Ibid, 2.
26. Ibid, 1.
27. Ibid, 10.
28. Ibid, 4–5.
29. Ibid.
30. 'Our History and Current Position,' *Ministry of Health Manatū Hauora*, 22 March 2012, http://www.health.govt.nz/about-ministry/ministry-business-units/Māori-health-business-unit/our-history-and-current-position.

31. *Guidelines He Ritenga Treaty of Waitangi Principles Health Audit Framework* (Tauranga, NZ: Bay of Plenty Health Board Hauora A Toi, 2004), 5, http://www.bopdhb.govt.nz/media/16348/AuditFrameworkGuidelines_Brown.pdf (accessed 9 July 2018).
32. Ibid, 10–15.
33. *Bay of Plenty District Health Board District Strategic Plan 2005–2015* (Tauranga, NZ: Bay of Plenty District Health Board Hauora a Toi, 2006), 7.

Chapter 12

1. *He Pou Oranga Tangata Whenua, Tangata Whenua Determinants of Health Framework* (Tauranga, NZ: Te Rūnanga Hauora o Te Moana a Toi, 2007), http://www.bopdhb.govt.nz/media/57182/hepouorangatangatawhenua.pdf (accessed 9 July 2018).
2. *Kōrero Mārama: Health Literacy and Māori. Results from the 2006 Adult Literacy and Life Skills Survey* (Wellington, NZ: Ministry of Health, 2010), 1, https://www.health.govt.nz/system/files/documents/publications/korero-marama.pdf (accessed 9 July 2018).
3. Ibid.
4. Ibid.
5. Ibid, iv.
6. 'Judith Amohaere Tangitu,' *Pū Kāea*, October–November, 2012, 13, http://tumekefm.co.nz/wp-content/uploads/2012/12/Pu-Kaea-Oct-Nov-2012-com.pdf (accessed 9 July 2018). The author also saw the citation for Judith Amohaere Tangitu at Whakatāne in 2015.
7. 'Official Opening of Whakatāne Campus Development,' *Scoop Independent News*, 5 December 2012, http://www.scoop.co.nz/stories/ED1212/S00022/official-opening-of-whakatane-campus-development.htm (accessed 9 July 2018).
8. The citation was seen by the author at Whakatāne in July 2016.
9. One example of this occurred with Granville Haami, an elderly Māori patient, who had a hip replacement operation at Whakatāne Hospital in September 2016. He had deep concerns for his own safety in the recuperating ward. 'Undergoing hip replacement surgery went without a hitch,' he said. But during his short recovery, he said 'the ward doctor yelled at me for no reason and nursing staff were uncaring to say the least'. The patient had to resort to speaking to the orderlies about the wrong medicine the nurse had given him. He never reported the incidents because he did not want to be fingered as rebellious by staff if he had to return for more treatment. Personal comment to the author by Granville Haami at Whakatāne, 2 October 2016.
10. 'Leading Together: Transforming He Pou Oranga Tangata Whenua Into Practice (Draft Version II – Version II)' (Bay of Plenty District Health Board, 17 April 2016), 5.
11. *BOPDHB Annual Plan 2015/16 Incorporating the Statement of Intent and Statement of Performance Expectations*, (Tauranga, NZ: Bay of Plenty District Health Board, September 2015), http://www.bopdhb.govt.nz/media/58478/bopdhb_2015-16_annual_plan.pdf (accessed 9 July 2018), 25.
12. 'Professor Angus Hikairo Macfarlane – Tertiary Teaching Excellence Teaching Profile' (*Ako Aotearoa*, October 2015), https://akoaotearoa.ac.nz/community/ako-aoteaora-academy-tertiary-teaching-excellence/resources/pages/professor-angus-hikairo-macfarlane-%E2%80%93-tertiary-teaching (accessed 9 July 2018).
13. 'Leading Together: Transforming He Pou Oranga Tangata Whenua Into Practice,' 2016, op. cit., 4–6.
14. Ibid.

SELECTED GLOSSARY

akuaku	cleanse
aroha	compassion, love
atawhai	care for, show kindness to
awhi	embrace
hapū	pregnant, sub-tribe
hauora	health
hunga	living, people
iwi	bones, tribe
kāhui	gathering
karakia	prayer, incantation
kaumātua	elder, elders
kawa whakaruruhau	cultural safety standards
kāwanatanga	governance
kōhanga	nest
kōhanga reo	language nest
kotahitanga	unity
kuia	elderly woman
kupenga	net, network
kupu arataki	introduction
māhaki	humble, meek, placid
mamae	pain
mana	authority,
mana atua	spiritual authority, connections to the spiritual world
mana tangata	recognition of personal authority, qualities and attributes
mana tupuna	acknowledgement of blood and kinship ties
mana whenua	authority over location, physical connection to the place of birth
manaaki	hospitality
Māori	indigenous people
mauri	life force
ngākau	heart

noa	free from tapu, unrestricted
oranga	health, living, wellbeing
paepae	orators' bench
Pākehā	New Zealander, non-Māori
pito	umbilical cord
pou kōkiri	cultural service providers
pou tūāpapa	core foundations
rangatiratanga	self-determination, soverignty
reo	language
rongoā	medicine
takohanga	obligation, responsibility
tangata whenua	people of the land
taonga	treasure
tapu	restriction, ritual separation, sacred
tikanga	protocol
tikanga rua	biculturalism
tohunga	traditional expert, specialist
toiora	wellbeing
tūpāpaku	deceased, dead body
tūroro	patient
urihaumate	patient (Mataatua dialect)
wairua	spirit
wairuatanga	spirituality, belief
whakanoa	to render a situation common or free from restriction
whakapapa	genealogy
whakawātea	to clear or free
whānau	family, give birth
whānau atawhai	caring family
whanaungatanga	relationship building

BIBLIOGRAPHY

Books, electronic references, journals, newspapers, reports, unpublished sources

A Fair Go for All? Rite Tahi Tatou Katoa? Addressing Structural Discrimination in Public Services, A Discussion Paper by the Human Rights Commission. Wellington, NZ: Human Rights Commission, July 2012. https://www.hrc.co.nz/files/2914/2409/4608/HRC-Structural-Report_final_webV1.pdf (accessed 9 July 2018).

'Auckland Area Health Board Policy on Biculturalism.' Auckland Area Health Board, Te Whānau Atawhai File, Amohaere Tangitu, 1990.

'Auckland Hospital Publication of Nursing Policy and Standards of Practice.' Auckland Healthcare, March 1994.

Auckland Sales and Hospital Endowments. Waitangi Tribunal Report 261. Wellington, NZ: Waitangi Tribunal, Department of Justice, 1991. https://forms.justice.govt.nz/search/Documents/WT/wt_DOC_68359805/Interim%20Report%20on%20Auckland%20Hospital%20Endowments.pdf (accessed 9 July 2018).

Barton, Pipi. '"A Kind of Ritual Pākehā Tikanga" – Māori Experiences of Hospitalisation: A Case Study.' Master of Philosophy in Nursing, Massey University, 2008.

'Basic Cultural Safety Aspects Stage Three.' Maori Health Services, Whakatāne Hospital, Pacific Health Ltd, 2004.

'Bay of Plenty District Health Board Hauora A Toi – Your DHB.' *Bay of Plenty District Health Board Hauora a Toi*, 14 August 2015. http://www.bopdhb.govt.nz/your-dhb/tauranga-hospital-centenary/m%C4%81ori-health/.

Bay of Plenty District Health Board District Strategic Plan 2005–2015. Tauranga, NZ: Bay of Plenty District Health Board Hauora a Toi, 2006.

Bay of Plenty District Health Board Māori Health Plan 2015/16. Tauranga, NZ: Bay of Plenty District Health Board, 2015. http://www.bopdhb.govt.nz/media/58163/bopdhb-maori-health-plan-2015-16.pdf (accessed 9 July 2018).

'Bay of Plenty District Health Board Position Statement – Health Inequalities.' Bay of Plenty District Health Board Hauora A Toi, n.d. http://www.bopdhb.govt.nz/media/33527/Position%20Statement%20Health%20Inequalities.pdf.

Best Health Outcomes for Māori: Practice Implications. Wellington, NZ: Medical Council of New Zealand, 2008.

'Bicultural Development in Nursing (Te Whakapakari Kakano Rua i Roto Mahi Tapuhi), Guidelines.' Review of the Preparation and Initial Employment of Nurses, National Action Group, 1991. http://www.moh.govt.nz/notebook/nbbooks.nsf/0/6df1f6d312be50d74c2565d700190096/$FILE/bicultural%20nursing.pdf (accessed 11 July 2018).

BOPDHB Annual Plan 2015/16 Incorporating the Statement of Intent and Statement of Performance Expectations. Tauranga, NZ: Bay of Plenty District Health Board, September 2015. http://www.bopdhb.govt.nz/media/58478/bopdhb_2015-16_annual_plan.pdf (accessed 9 July 2018).

Calder, Peter. 'A Rough Road towards Unity.' *New Zealand Herald*, 15 December 1990.
Camplin-Welch, Victoria. *Waitemata District Health Board Toolkit For Staff Working In A Culturally And Linguistically Diverse Health Environment*. Auckland, NZ: Waitemata District Health Board and Counties Manukau District Health Board, 2010. https://www.nzccp.co.nz/assets/Uploads/Cross-cultural-Toolkit-for-staff-CALD.pdf (accessed 11 July 2018).
Cartwright Inquiry, The Facts about the Cartwright Inquiry. http://www.cartwrightinquiry.com/ (accessed 23 March 2016).
Celebrating 100 Years of Innovation and Excellence, Tauranga Hospital 6 March 1914–2014. Tauranga, NZ: Bay of Plenty District Health Board, 2014. http://tauranga.kete.net.nz/documents/0000/0000/0448/Celebrating_100_years.pdf (accessed 9 July 2018).
Curtis, Toby. 'Letter to Dennis Pickup Chief Executive for Auckland Healthcare.' Te Whānau Atawhai Archive, Starship Hospital, 18 March 1994.
Dow, Derek A. *Maori Health and Government Policy 1840–1940*. Wellington, NZ: Victoria University Press, 1999.
Durie, Mason. *Maori Cultural Competencies for Health and Disability Advocates*. Wellingotn, NZ: Health and Disability Advocacy, Nga Kaitautoko, 2006. http://advocacy.hdc.org.nz/media/146523/m%C3%A4ori%20cultural%20competencies%20for%20health%20and%20disability%20advocates.pdf (accessed 10 October 2018).
———. 'Maori Health Transitions 1960–1985.' In *Huia Histories of Māori Ngā Tāhuhu Kōrero*, edited by Danny Keenan. Wellington, NZ: Huia Publishers, 2012.
———. *Mauri Ora: The Dynamics of Maori Health*. Auckland, NZ: Oxford University Press, 2001.
———. 'Pae Ora Maori Health Horizons.' Lecture paper presented at Te Mata o Te Tau Lecture Series, Massey University, 2009. http://www.manu-ao.ac.nz/massey/fms/manu-ao/documents/Pae%20Ora%20-%20Maori%20Health%20Horizons.pdf?B76AC0F2A1EF64CD377ADD13B162624E (accessed 9 July 2018).
———. 'The Treaty of Waitangi and Health Care.' *New Zealand Medical Journal*, no. 102 (1989).
———. *Whaiora: Maori Health Development*. 2nd ed. Auckland, NZ: Oxford University Press, 1998.
Employee Orientation and Information Booklet. Tauranga, NZ: Bay of Plenty District Health Board Hauora a Toi, 2014. http://www.bopdhb.govt.nz/media/41629/orientation-booklet-july-2014.pdf (accessed 12 July 2018).
Fifield, Anna. 'Amohaere Comes Home to Eastern Bay.' *Eastbay News*, 23 April 1998.
Guidelines for Cultural Safety. The Treaty of Waitangi and Māori Health and Wellbeing in Education and Psychological Practice. Wellington, NZ: New Zealand Psychologists Board, 2009. http://www.psychologistsboard.org.nz/cms_show_download.php?id=83 (accessed 11 July 2018).
Guidelines for Cultural Safety, the Treaty of Waitangi and Maori Health in Nursing Education and Practice. Wellington, NZ: Nursing Council of New Zealand, 2011. http://pro.healthmentoronline.com/assets/Uploads/refract/pdf/Nursing_Council_cultural-safety11.pdf (accessed 9 July 2018).
Guidelines He Ritenga Treaty of Waitangi Principles Health Audit Framework. Tauranga, NZ: Bay of Plenty Health Board Hauora A Toi, 2004. http://www.bopdhb.govt.nz/media/16348/AuditFrameworkGuidelines_Brown.pdf (accessed 9 July 2018).
Haami, Bradford. *Dr Golan Maaka Maori Doctor*. Auckland, NZ: Tandem Press, 1995.
Hauora o Te Moana Nui a Toi Bay of Plenty District Health Services Iwi Consultation Report. Tauranga, NZ: Bay of Plenty District Health Board, 2010.
'Haven of Peace.' *Rotorua Review*, 31 January 1995.
'He Kamaka Oranga Maori Health at ADHB.' *Nova Te Whetumarama, Te Pānui Mō Ngā Kaimahi a Te Toka Tumai*, July 2006.
He Pou Oranga Tangata Whenua, Tangata Whenua Determinants of Health. Tauranga, NZ: Te Rūnanga Hauora o Te Moana a Toi, 2007. http://www.bopdhb.govt.nz/media/57182/hepouorangatangatawhenua.pdf (accessed 9 July 2018).

'Healthy Communities Mauriora,' *Lakes District Health Board*, 13 June 2013. http://www.lakesdhb.govt.nz/Article.aspx?ID=2599.

'Hospital Pioneer Says Farewell.' *Nga Korero o Te Wa*, August 1994.

'Hospital Staff Lack "Bi-Cultural Understanding".' *Whakatāne Beacon*, 29 September 1998.

'Hunga Manaaki – Celebrating 10 Years of Service at Rotorua Hospital.' *Lakes District Health Board and Hunga Manaaki*, March 2007. http://www.lakesdhb.govt.nz/Resource.aspx?ID=7286.

'Judith Amohaere Tangitu Distinguished Fellow – Māori Health Sciences (Nursing).' *Pū Kāea*, October–November 2012.

Kapua, Terry. 'Cultural Competence Training, Te Whatumauri Hauora Whakatāne Hospital.' Te Whānau o Irākewa Māori Health Services, Whakatāne Hospital, November 2007.

Kearns, R.A., and J.R. Barnett. 'Happy Meals in the Starship Enterprise; Interpreting a Moral Geography of Health Care Consumption.' *Health and Place* 6, no. 2 (2000).

Keene, Lyndon. 'Working Against Racism.' *New Zealand Nursing Journal* 81 (August 1988).

Kingi, Te Kani. *Māori Mental Health: Past Trends, Current Issues, and Māori Responsiveness*. Wellington, NZ: Te Pūmanawa Hauora, Research School of Public Health, Massey University, 2005.

Kingi, Te Kani, Mason Durie, Hinemoa Elder, Rees Tapsell, Mark Lawrence, Simon Bennett. *Maea Te Toi Ora: Māori Health Transformations*. Wellington: Huia Publishers, 2018.

Knight, Stephenie. *Auckland Hospital Racism Intervention Project, A History*. Auckland: Race Relations Office and Auckland Hospital Board, 1989.

Kopae, Dianne. 'Health Initiatives Culturally-Friendly.' *Eastbay News*, 4 February 1999.

Kōrero Mārama: Health Literacy and Māori. Results from the 2006 Adult Literacy and Life Skills Survey. Wellington, NZ: Ministry of Health, 2010. https://www.health.govt.nz/system/files/documents/publications/korero-marama.pdf (accessed 9 July 2018).

Lange, Raeburn. 'Te Hauora Māori I Mua – History of Māori Health – Changing Health Onwards.' *Te Ara – the Encyclopedia of New Zealand*. Wellington, NZ: Ministry of Culture and Heritage, 5 May 2011, updated 1 June 2017. http://www.teara.govt.nz/en/te-hauora-maori-i-mua-history-of-maori-health/page-5 (accessed 12 July 2018).

McKegg, Alexandra. 'Cameron, Robina Thomson.' *The Dictionary of New Zealand Biography. Te Ara – the Encyclopedia of New Zealand*. Wellington, NZ: Ministry of Culture and Heritage, 6 June, 2013. http://www.TeAra.govt.nz/en/biographies/4c2/cameron-robina-thomson (accessed 9 July 2018).

Meredith, Paul. 'Urban Maori as "New Citizens": The Quest for Recognition and Resources.' In *Re Visioning Citizenship for the 21st Century, Proceedings of Re Visioning Citizenship for the 21st Century Conference*, edited by P. Havemann and G. Morgan. Hamilton: School of Law, University of Waikato, 2000.

Moore, Rina. 'The State of Maori Health.' *Te Ao Hou The New World*, no. 33 (December 1960): 6–11.

Moorfield, John C. *Maori Dictionary, Te Aka English–Maori, Maori–English Dictionary and Index*. New Zealand, 2016, 2003. Maoridictionary.co.nz.

'Mrs Te Amohaere Gardiner, Obituary'. *Te Ao Hou The New World*, no. 42, March 1963, http://teaohou.natlib.govt.nz/journals/teaohou/issue/Mao42TeA/c34.html (accessed 10 November 2014).

Mutu, Margaret. *The State of Maori Rights*. Wellington, NZ: Huia Publishers, 2011.

'New Zealand Health System Reforms.' *New Zealand Parliament*, 29 April 2009. http://www.parliament.nz/en-nz/parl-support/research-papers/00PLSocRP09031/new-zealand-health-system-reforms (accessed 7 November 2018).

Ngaropo, Amohaere G. 'Te Whānau Atawhai Integration of Te Whānau Atawhai with Greenlane and National Womens Hospitals, A Proposal to North Health.' Te Whānau Atawhai Archive, July 1994.

Ngaropo, Amohaere G., B.J. Anderson, and K. Way. 'Te Whānau Atawhai: A New Zealand Model For Supporting Indigenous Families With Children in Intensive Care.' Unpublished presentation, 1990.

Ngaropo, Pouroto. 'Ngā Pou Mana o Io Māori Health Services Integration into Toi Te Ora.' Māori Health Services Pacific Health, 11 July, 2003.

———. 'Nga Tikanga Whakahaere-a-Tangata Mo Toi Te Ora Cultural Safety. Aspects for Toi Te Ora When Engaging Tangata Whenua Mauriora. Maori Perspectives Relating to Cultural Safety.' Toi te Ora Community Health and Disability Services, Pacific Health, 2003.

'Official Opening of Whakatāne Campus Development.' *Scoop Independent News*. 5 December 2012. http://www.scoop.co.nz/stories/ED1212/S00022/official-opening-of-whakatane-campus-development.htm (accessed 9 July 2018).

'Our History and Current Position.' *Ministry of Health Manatū Hauora*. 22 March 2012. http://www.health.govt.nz/about-ministry/ministry-business-units/maori-health-business-unit/our-history-and-current-position.

Papps, Elaine, and Irihapeti Ramsden. 'Cultural Safety in Nursing: The New Zealand Experience.' *International Journal for Quality Health Care* 8, no. 5 (1996).

Pollock, Kerryn. 'Children's Homes and Fostering – Government Institutions.' *Te Ara – the Encyclopedia of New Zealand*. Wellington, NZ: Ministry of Culture and Heritage, 5 May 2011. http://www.TeAra.govt.nz/en/childrens-homes-and-fostering/page-2 (accessed 12 July 2018).

'Professor Angus Hikairo Macfarlane – Tertiary Teaching Excellence Teaching Profile.' *Ako Aotearoa*, October 2015. https://akoaotearoa.ac.nz/community/ako-aotearoa-academy-tertiary-teaching-excellence/resources/pages/professor-angus-hikairo-macfarlane-%E2%80%93-tertiary-teachi (accessed 9 July 2018).

Puao-Te-Ata-Tu (Day Break) The Report of the Ministerial Advisory Committee on a Māori Perspective for the Department of Social Welfare. Wellington, NZ: Department of Social Welfare, June 1986.

Ramsden, Irihapeti. 'Cultural Safety and Nursing Education in Aotearoa and Te Waipounamu.' Doctor of Philosophy thesis, Victoria University, 2002.

Report of the Committee of Inquiry into the Death at Carrington Hospital of Manihera Mansel Watene and Other Related Matters. Wellington, NZ: Department of Health, 1991. http://www.moh.govt.nz/notebook/nbbooks.nsf/0/6D27C1C11347822F4C2565D7000DEE34/$file/ Report_Committee_Inquiry_death_Carrington_Hospital.pdf (accessed 9 July 2018).

Richardson, Fran, and Lesley Macgibbon. 'Cultural Safety: Nurses' Accounts of Negotiating the Order of Things.' *Women's Studies Journal* 24, no. 2 (December 2010): 54–65.

'Situation Report Bicultural Development Auckland Hospital January 1990,' Te Whānau Atawhai Archive, January 1990.

'Starship Hospital Celebrates 21st Anniversary.' *New Zealand Herald*, 16 November 2012.

'Steps into the Future. Te Whānau Atawhai Developments to the Year 2000.' Te Whānau Atawhai Archive, February 1992.

Tamahori, Canon John. 'Maori Education.' *Te Ao Hou The New World*, 1 January 1972.

Tamahori, Canon John, and John Newman. 'Princess Mary Unit.' Whakatāne, Te Whānau Atawhai File, Amohaere Tangitu, 16 February 1990.

Tangitu, Amohaere Gardiner. 'Annual Report of the Maori Liaison Officer.' Auckland, NZ: Princess Mary Hospital, July 5, 1989.

Tangitu Ngaropo, Amohaere, and Naida Pou. 'He Kamaka Oranga Strategic Plan 1993/1994, Māori Health Management Developments to the Year 2000.' He Kamaka Oranga, 1994.

Tate, Henare Arekatera. *He Puna Iti I Te Ao Mārama A Little Spring in the World of Light*. New Zealand: Libro International, 2012.

———. 'Towards Some Foundations of a Systematic Māori Theology He Tirohanga Anganui Ki Ētahi Kaupapa Hōhonu Mō Te Whakapono Māori.' Doctorate of Philosophy, Melbourne College of Divinity, 2010.

Te Hauora O Te Moana Nui a Toi Pacific Health. Iwi Consultation. Whakatāne, NZ: Te Whatumauri Hauora Whakatāne Hospital, 2005.

'Te Pou Whatukura Cultural Practice Manual A Guide for Clinicians and Staff.' Mai i Nga Kuri a Wharei ki Tihirau Regional Maori Health Services. Bay of Plenty District Health Board, 2013.

'Te Pou Whatukura Cultural Practice Manual A Guide for Clinicians and Staff.' Bay of Plenty District Health Board, Edition Six, 2013.

'Te Tokotoko Poutiriao Te Whānau O Irākewa Staff Orientation Manual.' Bay of Plenty District Health Board, Whakatāne, 2007.

Te Whanau Atawhai, A New Initiative in Health Provision. Auckland, NZ: Te Whānau Atawhai, 1993.

Te Whanau Atawhai Annual Report – 1992. Auckland, NZ: Starship Hospital, October 1992.

'Te Whānau Atawhai Committee Meeting 16 March 1994.' Auckland, NZ: Te Whānau Atawhai Archive, Starship Hospital, 16 March 1994.

'Te Whānau Atawhai Meeting Minutes 9 September 1992.' Auckland, NZ: Te Whānau Atawhai Archive, Starship Hospital, 9 September 1992.

'The Cartwright Report.' *Cartwright Inquiry, The Facts About the Cartwright Inquiry*, 5 August 1988. http://www.cartwrightinquiry.com/?page_id=105 (accessed 23 March 2016).

Way, Karena. 'Leading Together: Transforming He Pou Oranga Tangata Whenua Into Practice (Draft Version II – Version II).' Bay of Plenty District Health Board, 17 April 2016.

'Whānau Accommodation – Te Whare Awhina.' *Starship Child Health*, 2015. https://www.starship.org.nz/patients-and-families/whats-at-starship/places-to-stay/whanau-accommodation-te-whare-awhina/.

Whittle, Patrick Michael. 'Darwinism and the Nature of Māori.' *MAI Review*, no. 3, 2009.

Whitwell, Shirely. 'Choice in Māori Health Service.' *Eastbay News*, 28 November 2002.

Interviews

Sir Toby Curtis
Ron Dunham
Sir Wira Gardiner
Lani Mārama
Dr John Newman
Pouroto Ngaropo
Amohaere Tangitu
Phyllis Tangitu
Heather Thompson
Karena Way

AUTHOR'S BIOGRAPHY

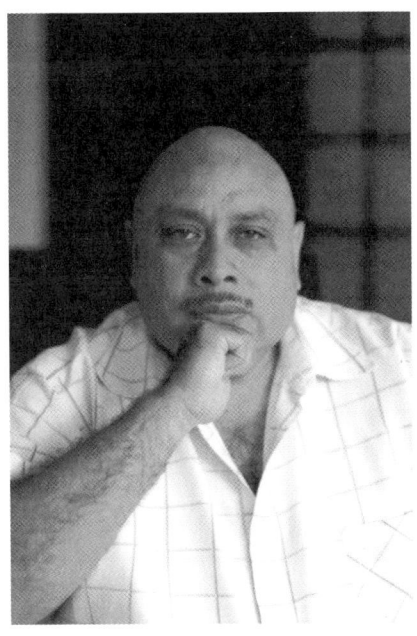

Bradford Haami is Ngāti Awa and lives in Auckland, New Zealand. He is an accomplished Māori writer with added experience in the television and film world. His passion for storytelling and expertise in Māori culture has seen him produce exploratory works on mātauranga Māori, Māori history and, more recently, Māori biography. His book *True Red: The Life of an ex-Mongrel Mob Gang Leader* (2004) captured audiences all over the world, selling unprecedented numbers of books, while *Ka Mau Te Wehi: Taking Haka To The World* (2013) (The life of Bub and Nen Wehi) won the 2013 Ngā Kupu Ora Best Māori Biography of the Year Award. Recently he published *The River of the Water of Life: A Biography of Ihaka 'Ike' Samuels* (2016) about a Māori missionary to Papua New Guinea and the very pertinent *Urban Māori: The Second Great Migration* (2018). He has also written for critically acclaimed television productions and has acted as a consultant to numerous local and international drama, documentary and feature films over the past two decades. His services were important to the making of the formidable *Mataku* series, *Tracker*, *Kiingitanga: The Untold Story* and, more recently, *Mahana*. 'My interest in storytelling is primarily based on the power of the story – whether in an oral form, a written form, a documentary or as a cinematic film – to convey a message that will stimulate conversation and ultimately transform hearts, minds and communities.'

INDEX

Bold typeface indicates photographs.

A

Ahomiro, Aronia 45, 64, **74**, 99, **153**, **156**
Auckland District Health Board 106, 109
Auckland Hospital 8, 10, 38, 46, 47, 56, 62– 63, 68, 83, 91, 93,
    98–102, 104, 106–107, 109, 116, 119, 143, **154**

B

Bastion Point 38
Bay of Plenty District Health Board 128, 135
bicultural 37, 39, 42, 57, 58, 85, 88, 90–91, 100–101, 103, 104, 109,
    114, 117, 126, 140
biculturalism 40, 55–57, 86, 89, 102–103, 106, 108, 115, 126, 130, 146

C

Cameron, Nurse Robina (Kamerana) 19
Carrington Polytechnic 36
Cowie, Rev. John 19
cultural safety 2, 8, 52, 58, 75, 81, 86–87, 103–104, 108–109, 115, 118,
    129, 130, 134, 138, 140, 146, 147
Curtis, Te Pere 62, 64, 72, **74**, 79–81

D

Dewes, Rev. Eru Potaka 41, 62, 64, **154**
Downes, Whakapūmautanga 113, 117, 126
Dunham, Ron 119, 121, 125, 128
Durie, Dr Mason 13, 40, 85, 86, 87, 101, 130

E

Eastbay Health Board 121, 123, 124, 126, 128

F

Futter, Mary (Mary Hackett) 37–38, 41, 57, 98, 131, **162**

G

Gardiner, Amohaere 16, 19, **19**, 20, 99
Gardiner, Tamehana 16–18, 20, **20**, 21, 23, 27, 29, 33
Grant, John 35
Gray, Ruby 62, 64, 98, 109, **156**
Greenlane Hospital 104–106, 107

H

Harawira, Titewhai 38, 42, 86
Head, Joan 41
He Kamaka Oranga 107–109
Hirsch, Wally 38
Hui Whakaoranga (1984) 86, 89
Hunga Manaaki 114–115, 117–119, **159**

I

institutional racism 35, 38, 39, 58

J

Jackson, Janet 41, 42

K

Kaa, Rev. Hone 9, 62, 64, 68, 81, 101
Kāhui Kaumātua 61, 63–73, **74**, 77–78, 81, 84, 85, 88, 91–93, 103,
    109, 112–115, 123–124, 126–127, **127**, 143, 144, **160**
kaiatawhai team 98, 106
Kawa Whakaruruhau, *see* cultural safety
Kereopa, Hohepa 119, 122, **123**
Kiriwera 22, 23–25

L

Lakeland Health 111, 112–114, 116–117
Lakes District Health Board 112, 113, 116, 117

M

Maaka, Dr Golan 25, 49
Malcolm, Joe Te Pōroa 112, 117
Māori Health 40, 86, 88, 91, 93, 101, 105, 107, 109, 113–116, 127,
    129, 131, 133–135, 140
Māori Women's Welfare League 85, 89
Mater Private Hospital 76
Medical Grand Round 94
Mihinui, Bubbles 114, 117
Morreau, Johan 118

INDEX

N

National Women's Hospital 104–105, 107
Newman, Dr John 44, 66, 88–90
Ngā Pou Mana o Io 131–134, 149
Ngaropo, Pouroto (Nicholas) 33, 72, 122, 124, 126, 127, 128, 131–133, **158, 159, 160**
Ngaropo, Samuel (Sam) 29, 32, 33, 34, 137
Ngaropo, Samuel Tawio 31

P

Pacific Health 127, 129, 134, 135
Pihama, Ann 109
Plunket 33
Pou (Glavish), Naida 107–108
Pou Taratu Senior Manager Māori Health 127
Powell, George 18, 19
Princess Mary Hospital 7, 37, 41, 45, 47, 62–63, 90, 97, 105, 131, **152**
Puao-Te-Ata-Tu Report 35, 39–40

Q

Queen Victoria Māori Girls College 19

R

race relations 38, 40, 86–87
racism 35, 38, 39, 40, 41, 56, 58, 72, 87
Raerino, Te Rame 30
Raharuhi, Gunner 112, 117
Ramsden, Irihapeti 52, 86–87
Rangihau, John 35, 36
Renata, Whareraupō 19
rongoā, *see* rongoā Māori
rongoā Māori 17, 70–71
Rotorua Hospital 111, 112, 114, 115, 116, 118, 119

S

Scott, Bob 38
Sharples, Dr Pita (Peter) 9, 38
Starship Hospital 47, 64, 90, 93, 99, 101, 102, **154, 155, 157, 158**
St Helen's National Women's maternity hospital 30, 33

T

Tamahori, Canon John 63–64, 72, 91–92, 98, 106, **154**
Tangitu, Cody 18, 26–28
Tangitu, Mihipeka (Mary) 18, 117, 126, **158**
Tangitu, Phyllis 99, 115, 116
Tāpuke, Bill 64, 91, 98, **156**

Te Arawa Health Authority 116
Te Arawa Trust Board 20
Te Atatū North 33, 34
Te Kupenga o Irākewa 126, 127
Te Mana Hauora o Te Arawa 112–113, 116, 120
Te Pou Kōkiri 127
Te Roopu Kai Ārahi Ki Te Ora 56, 57, 58, 101
Te Rūnanga Hauora o Te Moananui a Toi 138
Te Rūnanga o Te Moananui o Toi 128
Te Wānanga o Raukawa 85, 130
Te Whānau Atawhai 3, 64, 85, 91, 93–94, 97–100, **102**, 103–105, 106–109, 113–116, 144, **156**, **157**
Te Whānau o Irākewa 127, **127**, 129, 131, 134, 135
Te Whānau o Waipareira Trust 34, 107
Te Whare Awhina 47, *see also* Starship Hospital
Treaty of Waitangi 40, 56, 57, 86, 90, 102–103, 108–109, 129, 135
Tuoro, Mavis 64, 98
Turei, John 46, 62, 64

U

Umutahi 30, 32, 122

V

Vercoe, Bishop Whakahuihui 133
Vercoe, Charlie 119
Viliamu, Ake 73

W

Waikato District Health Board 112
wairua (wairuatanga) 13, 17, 49, 62, 68–69, 77, 81, 85, 86, 124, 134, 137, 149
Walker, Dr Ranginui 9, 38
Wallace, Mahia 56, 62, 64, 72, 98
Way, Karena 38–39, 41, 50, 56, 101, 102–103, **156**
Whakatāne Hospital 26, 29, 122, 127–129, 135, 139
Whānau House (Princess Mary Hospital) 44, 45, 47
Whānau Room (Starship Hospital) 47, 64, 91, 97, **157**
Wharepaia 42
Wikiriwhi, Doc 57, 62, 64, 68, 109
Williams, Brownie 45, 62, 64, **74**, 97, 98–99, 102, **153**